How Technology Is Changing Human Behavior

How Technology Is Changing Human Behavior

Issues and Benefits

C. G. Prado, Editor

Foreword by Rossana Pasquino

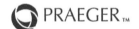 PRAEGER™

An Imprint of ABC-CLIO, LLC

Santa Barbara, California • Denver, Colorado

Library of Congress Cataloging-in-Publication Data

Names: Prado, C. G., editor.
Title: How technology is changing human behavior : issues and benefits /
    C. G. Prado, editor ; foreword by Rossana Pasquino.
Description: Santa Barbara, California: Praeger, an Imprint of ABC-CLIO, [2019] |
    Includes index.
Identifiers: LCCN 2018057360 | ISBN 9781440869518 (hardcopy) | ISBN
    9781440869525 (eBook)
Subjects: LCSH: Information technology—Social aspects. | Social
    media—Social aspects. | Identity (Psychology) | Human behavior.
Classification: LCC HM851 .H689 2019 | DDC 303.48/33—dc23
LC record available at https://lccn.loc.gov/2018057360

ISBN: 978-1-4408-6951-8 (print)
        978-1-4408-6952-5 (ebook)

23 22 21 20 19   1 2 3 4 5

This book is also available as an eBook.

Praeger
An Imprint of ABC-CLIO

ABC-CLIO, LLC
147 Castilian Drive
Santa Barbara, California 93117
www.abc-clio.com

This book is printed on acid-free paper ∞

Manufactured in the United States of America

Contents

Foreword

Rossana Pasquino

There are no passengers on spaceship earth. We are all crew.
—Marshall McLuhan

I have lived through a period in which fervor for technology widely changed teaching, learning, sport, and, in general, entertainment. I wrote my master's thesis using a personal computer that occupied my whole writing desk and was connected to an old-fashioned printer only capable of producing 100 black-and-white pages in a couple of hours. As a gift for my master's degree, I received from my parents a mobile telephone able only to call and to send 100 free text messages per month, with limited characters per message.

Today, 13 years later, everyone has a smartphone able to Google, pay bills, and "like" pages and the "status" of unknown people overseas. I can print hundreds of pages per minute using a superthin and light laptop, or so-called ultrabook, or via Bluetooth with my smartphone.

As a professor—or, more generally, as one of the knowledge holders—I feel the need to improve the learning experience for everyone by using methods alternative to traditional chalk and blackboard. In our athenaeum, active learning is spreading out, both to impart crucial knowledge and to assess understanding. We need to keep student audiences alert during lessons, and to gain their approval of our teaching—a sort of instant "like." At the end of a lesson, for example, many professors are using the "kahoot" method (www.kahoot.com). With a private account, professors can create on an online platform different learning games (known as kahoots) with multiple-choice questions regarding the topic of the lesson. The format and number of questions are entirely up to the professor, who has to indicate, when the kahoot is created, the right answers to the posed questions. Students answer the questions on their own smartphones (after having subscribed to the specific kahoot with their personal student pins) while the quiz is displayed on a shared screen. No worries about how many students have a smartphone; 100 percent of them do, and a very high percentage of them have power banks to be sure not to run out of battery power.

When the kahoot is finished, the answer statistics can be projected immediately on the screen, and the discussion between professor and students can begin. Professors can download the answers in an Excel file and can record and analyze them any time in the future. They can even assign kahoots as mandatory homework. The best students receive a bonus for their kahoots performance, which will increase their final exam scores. In this "learning gamification," everyone seems to receive his or her own recompense.

I also started wheelchair fencing five years ago, using an electrical saber. Thanks to weapon electrification, it is possible to register touches to a valid target with a light through an electric circuit. The referee has to indicate which fencer scores the point when both signals of the players light up by analyzing the movements that composed the last fencing phase. The decision is based on the concept of Right of Way, which gives the point to the fencer who had priority, and this can be gained in different ways. Of course, the referee could make the wrong decision, particularly when there were no lights to highlight the hits (while both fencers yell to acknowledge the point). Very recently, video refereeing has been introduced, with the same principle of the Video Assistant Referee in football. A video consultant is able to support or not support referees' decisions by video analysis, retracing the actions at issue. In this "gaming scientification," the fencer's rights are protected and suspense and tense atmosphere abolished.

Given my personal experience of this continuous trade-off between benefits provided by technological advancement in our lives and issues these improvements create in our approach to education, communication, sport, and human behavior, in general, I deeply appreciate the concerns this collection addresses.

Introduction: Technology Is Changing Us

C. G. Prado

Of all of technology's newly enabled devices, the one that seems to have the greatest impact on people is the smartphone. Replacing the highly useful but limited cell phone, the smartphone not only provides ready telephonic connectivity but also affords access to the Internet and has the capacity to run numerous "apps" that perform various tasks. The problem is that the use of smartphones has proven addictive, and like any addiction, it is affecting people in profound ways. The smartphone, though, is only one of many devices and capacities shaping and reshaping our behavior and, by doing so, shaping and reshaping us.

The end of the 20th century and the beginning of the 21st have seen technology advance impressively, and as its new procedures and devices are applied and employed, technology has not only improved life for many but has also increasingly influenced people by fostering practices that alter their lives and even their characters. A striking instance is the use of smartphones. No one who knows the amount of time spent by teenagers on their smartphones can doubt that use of some of the devices technological advancement has enabled affects people in significant ways, especially to the extent that using those devices engenders habitual behavior.

The most worrying aspect of engendered habitual behavior is its psychological impact. Habitual behavior regarding smartphones has received a good deal of attention. Many media and scholarly articles have been devoted to young people's excessive use of smartphones due to obsessive participation in social media sites and relentless texting. But there are less well-recognized instances of how use of smartphones, as well as tablets and laptops, is affecting people. One that I observed as a university professor, and deplore enough to have discussed in a radio interview, has to do with the reconception—or, perhaps better, the misconception—of learning and knowing.[1] Ready access to the Internet and search engines on smartphones, tablets, and laptops has resulted in many students reductively identifying knowledge with information. The outcome of this identification is a failure to understand why extensive instruction in subjects like history and geography is necessary when the data is readily available through use of Internet search engines. This consequence constitutes a serious failure on the part of students to grasp the difference between learning and comprehension, on the one hand, and mere acquisition and possession of data on the other. Because of this failure, students are impatient with and easily distracted from instructors' efforts to have them assimilate and integrate the material covered in lectures and coursework. Students have come to see that material as just so much data, as data far more easily accessed on the Internet than through what they now think of as tedious lectures and dreary textbooks. The result is that education is failing to edify them. Education is failing to give students assimilated understanding of conveyed material due to their perception and acceptance of the Internet as the repository of data they need not keep in their heads.

We are living in a time when technological advancement is not only outstripping the pace of its progression in previous eras but is also affecting many more aspects of our lives than ever before. One negative way technological advancement is affecting us is by making many jobs redundant and thus threatening to decrease employment to an extent that will leave millions of workers jobless. Against this, a positive way technological advancement is affecting us is by enabling impressive progress in various fields as diverse as space exploration and criminal investigation. But while we may delight in watching televised coverage of fly-bys inspecting Jupiter's satellites and following how DNA analysis expedites investigatory police work, the vast majority of us are, and will remain, observers with respect to employment of technological capacities like these. However, in the case of smartphones and employment of their capacities, we are thoroughly engaged participants.

Unquestionably, smartphones, tablets, and laptops offer us impressive capabilities. Access to the Internet is the most notable, but even when smartphones fail to detect a signal or, along with pads and laptops, fail to get online because of lack of Wi-Fi, these devices can be used to read existing texts and reminders, to watch previously downloaded videos, to compose everything from memos to manuscripts, to browse through saved photos, to listen to favorite downloaded songs, to play one game or another, and to employ various apps that perform many other jobs. On the downside, exercise of these capabilities is attention demanding, time consuming, and distracting from what is going on in users' immediate personal and social environments.

My objective in this introductory essay is to discuss what I believe to be the most serious consequence of obsessive smartphone use, a consequence I have labeled "loss of personal priority." The articles or chapters that follow this introduction focus on a number of questions arising from the use of innovative devices and practices enabled by technological progress.[2] Contributors have pursued issues that especially concern them. My own concern centers on the growing, obsessive use of smartphones—use that is affecting a very large number of people in significant and, unfortunately, largely negative ways. As the nearly fanatical playing of video games by many demonstrates, there is also obsessive use of tablets and laptops, but the versatility of smartphones, and especially their easy portability, make them considerably more likely to prompt and support excessive use. Because of their handiness, smartphones are now as much a part of people's normal accoutrements as are wristwatches and wallets, and the ready availability of one's smartphone is deemed a practical necessity. But unlike wallets and wristwatches, smartphones encourage and support compulsive usage to an alarming degree.

Discussion of excessive use of smartphones by experts and journalists runs the gamut from physical effects through psychological effects to social effects. For example, with respect to physical effects, excessive smartphone usage produces what is called "text-neck." This condition results from the bowed-head posture that using smartphones involves, which increases the gravitational pull on users' spinal cords.[3] As for social and psychological effects, Alan Popescu observed that "75 percent of Americans believe their smartphone usage doesn't impact their ability to pay attention . . . according to the Pew Research Center, and about a third of Americans believe that using phones in social settings actually contributes to the conversation." Popescu adds that contrary to these views, experts maintain that what he calls the "always-on" behavior of smartphone users actually "causes us to remove ourselves from our reality."[4]

What Popescu calls "always-on behavior" is an attitudinal disposition, a disposition to engage with one's smartphone continuously. Enactment of this disposition is evident all around us in how, for too many users, smartphone alerts take precedence over whatever else they may be doing. As I am sure readers also do, I regularly witness serious business and personal exchanges interrupted by one or another of the parties involved responding to a smartphone's cascade of syncopated noise or silent vibration. Their attention then focuses on the smartphone screen or they answer the call and mutter the now hackneyed phrase, "I have to take this." In the many cases I have noted, I do not recall a single instance when the alerting smartphone was simply turned off or ignored rather than the call being answered or the screen being checked.

Naturally, some smartphone calls may well be quite important, such as for physicians on duty and similar cases, but given the number of users and their average status, pressing calls are decidedly in the minority. In any case, the fact is that regardless of the possible importance of incoming calls, users now regularly give their smartphones priority over whatever else may be going on. This is what I am calling a loss of personal attention priority. The loss occurs when smartphone users come to regularly yield to their smartphones' alerts rather than stick to their own priorities in conversations and other activities. This loss of attention priority is essentially individuals forfeiting authority over their own intentions and objectives. It is a forfeiture of personal control to the extent that smartphone alerts prompt immediate responses regardless of what else users may be saying or doing or about to say or do.

The loss of attention priority has serious repercussions, the most serious being that automatic prioritization of smartphone alerts inescapably lowers the priority of whatever else users are up to. In terms of interactions with others, answering a smartphone or even just checking its screen in the middle of a personal or business conversation cannot be anything other than allowing the alert to supersede the interrupted exchange. Against this, ignoring a smartphone alert confirms the priority of the interaction taking place, no doubt to the gratification of the user's interlocutor or interlocutors.

Where a priority shift from ongoing exchanges to smartphones is most disturbing to interlocutors, and most obvious to bystanders, is when the interrupted conversation is a thorny business one or an intimate tête-à-tête between partners or spouses. In these cases, interlocutors tend to consider the smartphone taking priority as a lessening of the importance of their ongoing exchange and likely as a personal slight. We have all witnessed looks of impatience and of annoyance on the part of interlocutors when someone they are speaking with interrupts the exchange to answer or check a smartphone. However, indicative of the progression of smartphone prioritization is that smartphone users are increasingly responding to their interlocutors' smartphone interruptions by checking their own smartphones.

The importance of loss of attention priority amounts to what it is not too much to describe as self-diminishment. Loss of attention priority is self-diminishment in that giving smartphone alerts priority as described is incontestably the result of addiction, and succumbing to addiction is a lessening of the self to the extent that it reduces individuals' ability to pursue their own intentions and abide by their own decisions. To make matters worse, loss of attention priority does not affect only smartphone users themselves; rather, it has substantial repercussions for others as well. The most notable instance of this is the negative impact of parental smartphone distraction on children.

Erika Christakis reviewed how consistent use of smartphones not only distracts parents from day-to-day domestic care of their young children, but it also introduces highly incapacitating factors into the children's development. Christakis observed that distraction due to use of smartphones results in "continuous partial attention" that impairs children's development by interrupting the "cueing system, whose hallmark is responsive communication."[5] This cueing system has to do with how infants mimic parental facial expressions and, later, parental comments. The mimicking is integral to the process of children learning how to express themselves both facially and linguistically. Deborah Fallows, herself a linguist, anticipated Christakis's concern, reviewing studies that indicated how parental overuse of smartphones negatively affects children's learning of language due to lack of focused communicative interaction between parent and child.[6] This negative outcome of excessive smartphone use is very serious because it adversely affects children's development as persons and as social entities.

The unavoidable question is this: What is it about smartphones that makes their use addictive and leads to loss of attention priority? Answering this question begins with understanding that use of smartphones is not only a matter of intended or anticipated communication. That is, users are not only prompted to answer incoming calls and to make outgoing ones. That was the case with the use of cellphones, but smartphones effected an extraordinary change by enabling access to the Internet and social media sites. Where cellphones enabled exchanges with particular individuals, smartphones enable users to check their e-mail accounts, to log on to websites that permit and invite postings and so let users participate in ongoing exchanges with thousands of others, to review held opinions on subjects that interest them on blogs and other discursive or broadly conversational websites, and to express their own views to huge audiences on those same websites. This access and what it entails reveals that there are two aspects to smartphone use. First, there is the *communicative* aspect, which has to do fairly narrowly with expecting and receiving calls from, and making calls to, particular persons. The second aspect can be described as the *participatory* aspect. This participatory aspect covers Internet access to and engagement in a wide range of social media and other discursive sites. The participatory aspect also covers employment of Internet search engines prompted by issues or questions arising in discussions occurring in physical or digital space.

The combined communicative and participatory aspects of smartphone use are the springboard for addictive use. Exercise of both constitutes potentially habitual behavior that easily becomes addictive. William Wan characterized the process of smartphone addiction by drawing a perceptive parallel with B. F. Skinner's experimentation with conditioning. Wan put the central point this way:

> In the 1950s, Skinner began putting [pigeons] in a box and training them to peck on a piece of plastic whenever they wanted food. Then the Harvard psychology researcher rigged the system so that not every peck would yield a tasty treat. It became random—a reward every three pecks, then five pecks, then two pecks. The pigeons went crazy and began pecking compulsively for hours on end. . . . Fast forward six decades. We have become the pigeons pecking at our iPhones.[7]

But what is it that "pecking at our iPhones" yields? That is, what is the incentive that prompts compulsive use of smartphones? For Skinner's pigeons it was the possibility of a tasty treat. What moves smartphone users?

There are three different incentives that drive excessive attention to and use of smartphones. One incentive is in line with the communicative aspect of smartphone use and basically is gratification for being addressed, for being the object of someone's attention. A second incentive is in line with the participatory aspect of smartphone use and is essentially gratification for belonging, for being part of a group. The third incentive, also in line with the participatory aspect, is gratification at "being in the know," for resolving issues and questions. The first incentive results in smartphone users giving primacy to incoming calls. The second incentive results in smartphone users regularly accessing and developing allegiances to Internet and social media websites that satisfy their broadly cultural and sociopolitical preferences and inclinations. The third incentive results in smartphone users persistently using the Internet to find or check information.[8]

Taken together, these incentives provide a strong impetus for ever-greater use of and dependence on smartphones; and given human nature, that dependence inevitably morphs into addiction—and with that comes loss of personal attention priority. Smartphone alerts then take priority over any ongoing exchange, and the sheer presence of users' smartphones provokes them to log on to various sites, overriding whatever else they may be doing.

Provocation to access the Internet on a smartphone is difficult to pin down concisely. It seems to be a matter of the smartphone just being *there*, but the smartphone is not there as a device; it is there as an inviting portal, as an entryway. To appreciate how this works, imagine that you have just stepped out of a room in which captivating conversations are taking place. The smartphone is like the open door through which you left the room, and through which you can reenter the room. The conversations remain ongoing, and through the smartphone portal, you can again continue being part of them. In this way, the smartphone is a constant invitation to engage in whatever is going on in digital space.

As I have indicated, there have been many warnings about excessive smartphone use. The impact of these alerts has been and continues to be marginal. The smartphone is almost certainly the single most influential product of technological advancement, and as such, it is having the greatest effect on people and their habits. It is very, very difficult to imagine a significant reduction in smartphone use occurring anytime soon, if at all. In this respect, technological advancement has decidedly changed us, and the consequences of the change are yet to be tracked, assessed, and dealt with.

To close this brief introduction, I want to stress that the articles that follow are not about technology per se. The articles are about what technology enables and some of the consequences of that enablement—consequences that are primarily practices that change people's behavior and, in doing so, remold who they are. The hard question technological enablement raises is this: When do the changes that new devices foster make people and their lives better, and when they do the opposite? Contributors to this collection approach this question from different backgrounds, interests, and expertise. My objective as editor was to gather diverse perspectives on technological enablement, but the aim of the collection is not to convince readers of one view or another of the consequences of technological enablement. The aim of the collection is to prompt readers to think seriously about the various issues considered.

Notes

1. C.G. Prado, CFRC-FM, "What on Earth Is Going On . . . With the Digital Age," Episode 2, May 11, 2018, available as a podcast at www.woegoshow.com.

2. There are many other relevant issues aside from those discussed below, far too many for us to have dealt with in this collection. For instance, consider: https://www.technologyreview.com/s/608248/biased-algorithms-are-every where-and-no-one-seems-to-care/. Also consider: https://www.digitaltrends.com /cool-tech/algorithms-of-oppression-racist/. My thanks to Lisa Portmess for alerting me to these two sites. See also "Nowhere to Hide," Leaders Section, *Economist*, September 9, 2017, p. 11; "Keeping a Straight Face," Science and Technology Section, *Economist*, September 9, 2017, pp. 73–75; and Deb Riechmann, "Rapidly Advancing Face-Mapping Technology 'Could Create Real Chaos' in Era of Fake News," *Globe and Mail*, July 3, 2018, Section A, p. 2.

3. Adam Popescu, "Keep Your Head Up: How Smartphone Addiction Kills Manners and Moods," *New York Times*, January 25, 2018.

4. Ibid.

5. Erika Christakis, "The Dangers of Distracted Parenting," *The Atlantic*, July/August 2018, p. 12.

6. Deborah Fallows, "Papa, Don't Text," *The Atlantic*, July/August 2013, p. 23.

7. William Wan, "Rebel Developers Are Trying to Cure Our Smartphone Addiction—With an App," Health and Science Section, *Washington Post*, June 17, 2018.

8. For example, www.wikipedia.org and www.imdb.com are websites regularly accessed during conversations.

CHAPTER ONE

The Robotization of Everything

Lawrie McFarlane

In this chapter, I examine the potential impact of robotization, principally on employment but also on some other aspects of human interaction, specifically sexual relations, patient care, and distance education. The advent of intelligent machinery has been termed the fourth industrial revolution, the preceding three being the original 19th-century version; the commodity revolution of the early 20th century, which brought widespread access to new consumer goods like the telephone and the automobile; and the digital revolution, which began in the 1980s and continues to this day. The development of robotics and intelligent machinery, however, belongs in a class of its own. Not only does it offer new technologies that were previously unavailable, but it has also begun to blur the lines between the animate (humans) and the inanimate (machines). It is with this fourth industrial revolution that I am concerned.

A recent study by the McKinsey Global Institute found that in the majority of occupations, at least one-third of the work is automatable.[1] That translates into 800 million jobs worldwide. In the United States, according to McKinsey, 70 million Americans may lose their jobs to robotics, artificial intelligence, and machine learning by the year 2030. The equivalent figure for Canada is around eight million jobs—in both cases, roughly 30 percent of the workforce.

It might be thought that the introduction of such revolutionary technologies would generate sufficient new employment opportunities to compensate for jobs lost. But that is not the conclusion of the study. Its authors estimate that around 365 million new jobs will indeed be created across the globe, yet that is less than half the number required to preserve the status quo. In effect, hundreds of millions will have to retrain for different forms of employment, and this is not a simple proposition. The main impact of robotization will, at least initially, fall on those least able to cope with a career change—employees who perform physical or routine tasks and those whose employment requires little training or education beyond high school level. As it is implausible to suppose that all, or even the majority, of these workers will successfully make the transitions required, we must assume that many will be forced to leave the workforce entirely.

The first proposition I advance, then, is that robotization is almost certain to have a disastrous effect on employment. But this is a contentious claim. The original industrial revolution had the opposite effect. The economic growth it gave rise to more than compensated for job loss in some isolated sectors. Prior to the revolution, most national economies were agrarian in nature. Economic growth, measured both in GDP and employment rates, had moved at a glacial rate for centuries. But in the United Kingdom, where full-scale mechanization of the workplace had its beginnings, that suddenly changed. Between 1800 and 1900, Britain's GDP increased by more than 600 percent. By 2000, average per capita income in fully industrialized countries was 52 times greater than in nonindustrial nations.[2]

There was indeed considerable loss of jobs. The farming sector in particular was hard hit—understandably so as it represented the principal employment opportunity prior to industrialization. And, no doubt, many workers who could not adapt to factory life and the increased presence of machinery were displaced and their lives greatly disrupted However, it is beyond dispute that the first industrial revolution not only enormously increased output and generated more jobs than were killed but also fueled a growth in incomes and in national wealth that facilitated better health care, public education, and social services. It might be said that the social safety net we take for granted in developed countries owes its origin to industrialization. In short, the benefits outweighed the costs.

It is my intent to argue that robotization will not have these positive effects. It may increase output, and it may also relieve humans of the need to undertake some of the more dangerous forms of employment like coal mining. But the overall cost will be massive job loss and serious impacts on human welfare. To support this proposition, it is necessary to consider the sheer scale of what may lie ahead. The fields of employment most immediately threatened are those in which repetitive tasks predominate.

Plans are underway, for instance, to build a truck highway from Mexico to Canada used entirely by automated vehicles. The monetary benefits are obvious. By law, human truckers in the United States must take an eight-hour break each day. In Canada, the daily log-off time is 10 hours. Robots, of course, require no such time-outs. Many transit rail systems are already driverless, and fully automated cars are already making an appearance (though not without incident). But it is a virtual certainty that robotization, as it grows in sophistication, will not be confined to forms of employment that depend largely on unskilled labor.

Here a further consideration arises. The machines introduced during the first industrial revolution, by and large, had limited application. In other words, they were narrowly task specific. And although they were constantly improved or replaced by more advanced technologies, their scope remained relatively confined. It was possible, in short, for humans and machines to coexist, as the latter were no match for humans across a wide range of tasks. But will we retain this advantage once robotization takes off? Artificial intelligence is continually expanding its reach, in the process encroaching ever further on behavior we once thought uniquely human. The robotization project is not a force multiplier whose objective is to supplement human labor. Its purpose—and increasingly its capability—is to displace humans.

This last point requires further elaboration. The rate at which artificial intelligence is progressing far exceeds our experience with mechanization during the first industrial revolution. From a standing start in the late 1940s, when the first programmable computers were built, we now have machines that can compose tolerable prose, write original music, and beat chess masters. They can fly aircraft, steer ships, and take over a range of household tasks. They can even produce paintings that art experts cannot distinguish from the "real" thing. It is becoming increasingly difficult to imagine what they might one day accomplish. But this is precisely the point. How long can human labor compete when artificial intelligence shows every sign of being able to match or exceed our performance across a wide range of what were once considered human monopolies?

There is also the possibility that as robots expand their powers, they will begin to retool themselves. That is to say, they will learn as they go, continually adding to their capabilities. Google's AlphaZero computer program taught itself chess in four hours and went on to beat a champion chess program. And they will not only expand their own capabilities. It must be expected that they will learn to build more advanced machines than human designers might have thought of. That is to say, current generations of artificial intelligence may give rise, on their own, to future generations. But reproduction, so far, has been solely an attribute of living things. Whether robotic regeneration should be considered a form of reproduction is a question I'm happy to leave to philosophers. However, if first-generation robots can build second-generation robots with extended powers, then the threat they pose to human employment grows exponentially.

It is necessary at this stage to consider a counterargument that some who favor robotization of the workplace have put forward. They accept that humans will indeed be replaced by machines in many worksites, but they suggest that, so long as the economy expands due to the greater productivity that smart machines offer, it should be possible to provide financial compensation to those workers who are laid off. Some social policy experts, for instance, have argued that governments should create a "basic income" that everyone of working age would receive. The idea is to ensure that unemployment does not lead to a loss of financial well-being.

But here it is necessary to introduce an observation about psychology. People need to work in order to preserve self-worth and create a sense of personal achievement. We need to be busy, and preferably in the pursuit of some task we find meaningful or rewarding. We also need to feel self-reliant, meaning we are able, through our labor, to put food on the table, raise a family, and (hopefully) generate savings for retirement. There is an old saying that found money is soon squandered. There is some truth in this. We place more value on wealth we earn through our own hard work than on money that comes easily. I raise this latter point for the following reason.

A paper published by the Australian Psychological Society in 2000[3] makes several useful observations, among them that work provides a sense of purposefulness and social contact, that employed people generally enjoy better mental health than those who are unemployed, that job loss in middle age is particularly damaging, and that research in Sweden[4] has shown considerable psychological and health strains associated with job loss. So far, the paper covers ground already well researched—the positive relationship between employment and personal well-being.

However, the authors go a step further. They note that attempts to offset with financial assistance the harm caused by job loss have not necessarily succeeded. This last point is noteworthy. The Swedish research suggests that merely guaranteeing people who lose their job a basic income does not compensate for the deprivation of personal dignity and self-worth. In effect, while a basic income, or some such mechanism, is undoubtedly better than nothing (whether it is affordable is another matter), what counts most is job retention. I will discuss at the end of this chapter what measures might be taken to counter the threat to human employment created by robotization and the spread of artificial intelligence.

But there is a second argument in favor of robotization, which is that although many jobs will undoubtedly be lost, in some instances that may be no bad thing. Do we really want humans digging coal in mines, inhaling dust, and putting their future health at risk? Is working as a prison guard in a supermax penitentiary a life-fulfilling occupation? Or how about cleaning up a radiation spill or working as a logger, well up on the list of the 10 most dangerous jobs? Does not the argument that humans need employment weaken when the form of employment concerned is potentially destructive?

I concede there is a case to be made here, though how we draw the line between acceptable employment and the overly dangerous variety, I have no idea. But at most this is a quibble. We may very well want to fence off some specific jobs as simply too threatening for humans to engage in if a robot can take over. But these are a tiny proportion of the various forms of employment. And here the principal argument against robotization must be restated. Humans need work, even if it is at times risky, tedious, or even dangerous. That a robot could do the work is not the issue. That people *need* to work is the point at stake.

But it is not only the threat of job loss that concerns me. The second proposition I wish to advance is that different kinds of human needs will also be negatively affected. Specifically, I want to look at the impact of artificial intelligence on sexual relations, patient care, and distance education. Beginning with the first of these—sexual relations—male and female sex robots with lifelike appearance and programmable behavior are beginning to make an appearance. Already there are brothels in several European countries that offer robots as an alternative to the "real" thing. That may be an exaggeration. So far, although top-of-the-line models can swivel their eyes, move their lips in synch with programmed answers to simple questions—"My name is Crystal" and so forth—they have no ability to move their limbs and perform more complex tasks like walking. They are basically lifeless dolls with small computer chips embedded that enable them to perform the simplest of tasks. However, it is certain this will not remain true for long. Some experts in the field predict the arrival of far more lifelike models that will be, behaviorally speaking, indistinguishable from humans without the help of a Blade Runner. These avatars would possess the power of speech and movement, the ability to maintain a conversation, and also a learning mode that would enable them to improve their performance, verbally and otherwise, over time.

It is not difficult to foresee the issues that may arise. Might we expect humans to find sex with a machine either preferable, or at any rate sufficiently adequate, that the need and desire to find a human mate declines? We already live in a time when relations between the sexes have grown strained. The #MeToo movement originated with evidence of gross sexual misbehavior by men in the entertainment and news industries. But allegations of toxic masculinity have escalated. While many of these allegations are true, some male managers are now avoiding their female colleagues for fear of career-ending accusations. The more widespread this form of stress becomes, the more robot companions may start to appear attractive. Robots may not be the perfect mate, but they might very well be safer.

Down this road lie several troubling scenarios. The implications for reproduction are evident. We already face a situation in which none of the developed countries maintains sustainable birth rates. In Japan, nearly half the men and women of marrying age say they have never had a romantic relationship with a member of the opposite sex (or the same sex) and have no great wish to try.[5] Add robot companions, and it would seem that things can only get worse. Physiotherapist Masayuki Ozak from Tokyo takes his silicon avatar out on dates (he carts "her" around in a wheelchair). He and his wife share a bed with young Mayu.[6] It does not appear to be an unreasonable inference that the very idea of reproduction may be in the process of acquiring a faintly passé aura.

Of course, there have always been forms of sexual interaction that were not aimed at reproduction. The world's oldest profession came into being to satisfy the urges, largely of men, whose purpose was not to produce a child. But the social stigma, not to mention legal constraints associated with prostitution, ensured that this would never become a genuine threat to the continuation of our species. The imminent introduction of sophisticated sex robots changes that prospect. Sexual relations have always been one of the main adhesives that bound men and women together. Now that adhesive is weakened by a new alternative that offers some of the same satisfactions with none of the concomitant responsibilities.

There is also the troubling issue of sexual aggression. Some manufacturers are programming their sex robots to put up a show of resistance when their owners, partners, despoilers—whatever we call them— demand sex. The objective, apparently, is to reward a tendency in some men toward aggression or worse. But is this really a behavior we want to encourage?

Unlike the other forms of social dislocation discussed in this chapter, the pending advent of sophisticated sex robots poses questions—and threats—that no other technological advance has come close to. We learned to live with mechanized factories. We welcomed horseless carriages. The cell phone, and likewise the Internet, while frequently disruptive (we now have a generation of young people ensconced in their parents' basements, texting friends instead of actually meeting them), have hugely advanced the dissemination of knowledge and information. But sex robots, through their capacity to offer an alternative to the most basic, and crucial, form of human interaction, represent an unprecedented peril. It would be an exaggeration to say there is an existential threat to our species here. No doubt human reproduction will continue.

But how men and women view each other, and the care and attention they extend to one another, may very well be altered for the worse. A population of undemanding avatars, built to satisfy their owners without requiring reciprocal compassion, seems likely to depreciate the value system that governs human relationships. Competition doesn't force prices up, it forces them down. An increase in supply doesn't raise prices, it lowers them. And the price that may be lowered here is the quantum of love and devotion men and women believe they owe each other.

Yet we cannot leave the issue there. Numerous studies have shown that a significant proportion of men are too shy or too socially inept to form lasting relationships with the opposite sex. The same, to a lesser extent, is true of women. Are they to be denied the opportunity of resorting to a mechanized companion? Likewise, many elderly men and women whose spouses have died find themselves in a position where it is difficult to meet a new partner. The same question arises: Don't they have a legitimate claim to some form of outlet? There are numerous situations where behavior that would be objectionable or damaging if engaged in broadly is tolerated in narrowly defined circumstances. Canadian law, for example, makes it an offense to assist in a suicide. Yet an exception is made for physician-assisted suicide in cases where a patient is in extreme discomfort and death is imminent. Unfortunately, it appears impossible to imagine a comparable regulatory regime that would outlaw general access to sex robots while permitting exceptions in the case of individuals whose personal circumstances preclude their finding a human mate.

I have no idea how the challenges and threats posed by sex robots can be resolved. But the time is not far off when we will be required to manufacture a solution.

I want to turn now to the impact of artificial intelligence on patient care. The general presumption to date has been that robotization represents a threat primarily to low-income, low skill–level jobs. However, there are opportunities for smart machines to carry out much more sophisticated tasks. Bond trading and some aspects of accounting are viable fields for the introduction of artificial intelligence. Computer algorithms have already demonstrated a superior ability to detect profitable patterns in large stock market databases.

But it is in patient care that some of the greatest opportunities—and dangers—exist. Computers can already scan laboratory test results and some diagnostic images not only far more rapidly but also with greater accuracy than humans. Robots have been designed that can diagnose several neurological disorders merely by "listening" to voice recordings from patients. They can also diagnose some forms of cancer with more precision than oncologists.[7] And the da Vinci robotic surgery system can assist in the removal of prostate tumors with fewer harmful side effects for the patient.[8]

In truth I see little real danger in these developments so far. It makes sense, for example, to augment the work of elderly surgeons whose hand control has diminished with robots that suffer no such ill effects. However, if we begin to see robots gaining a more extensive presence in hospital wards and long-term care facilities, I believe there is cause for concern. Patient care in its most essential aspects requires a degree of compassion and human contact. Machines may learn to mimic some of those interactions, but they are still machines. Yet the temptations will be enormous. Acute care nurses in the United States earn anywhere from $60,000 to $110,000 per year, pay and benefits included. But at least some of their work, and conceivably all of it, could be robotized. It will take no great advance to design intelligent machines that can give injections, detect fever or other symptoms, read physician instructions, and carry out other basic elements of patient care. Indeed, researchers at Rutgers University have constructed a "venipuncture robot" that uses near-infrared and ultrasound imaging to locate a usable vein and draw blood from it. This new technology makes it easier to extract samples from difficult patient groups, such as small children.[9] And robots don't need to be paid time and a half for working extra shifts.

It is also necessary at this point to admit into the debate some of the foibles that care providers exhibit, but machines do not. Nurses are more likely to take sick days or go on extended leave than most other classes of employee. The reasons are obvious. Patient care, particularly in intensive care wards like burn units, is immensely stressful. And this stress has only magnified as hospitals across North America have struggled to keep costs down. I can speak from personal experience here, both as a former deputy minister of health in British Columbia and as a CEO of the first regional health authority in Saskatchewan.

A brief history of the events leading up to cost cutting in acute-care facilities may be helpful. Between the late 1960s and the mid-1990s, Canada's federal and provincial governments, with a couple of exceptions, ran deficits every year, as did most Western countries, the United States included. This was a period of rapid growth in the size and scope of government. In Canada, total spending (provincial and federal combined) rose from 14 percent of GDP in 1960 to 53 percent in 1995. And those are inflation-adjusted numbers.[10] By the end of this period, several provinces were headed toward bankruptcy (Saskatchewan was rescued by a last-minute bailout from Ottawa), and government credit ratings had deteriorated significantly. Beginning in 1996 there was a concerted effort by most governments in Canada, federal as well as provincial, to turn the situation around. Inevitably the axe fell most heavily on health care as it represented around 40 percent of total public-sector spending.

Hospitals were targeted because they consumed the largest share of the health care budget. Same-day surgery was introduced (meaning the patient was not brought into the hospital the night before, as had long been the practice). Most surgeries were shifted to an outpatient basis, a change made possible, in part, by the introduction of laparoscopic surgery, which requires a minimal incision. Surgery patients who previously would have remained in the hospital for a week or more went home in a day or two. Mothers with a normal birth were sent home with their infants after 24 to 48 hours instead of the three- to five-day stay in years gone by. One result of these and other changes was a dramatic reduction in the number of hospital beds, both in total and per capita. In British Columbia there are, today, 30 percent fewer people in hospital beds than there were 15 years ago, and the province's population has grown over that period by nearly 20 percent. The same is true, in varying degrees, across the country. Among the 39 OECD countries, Canada is now close to the bottom in hospital beds per capita. In 2015 Canada had 2.61 beds per 1,000 people. Japan, at the top of the list, had 13.17. The United States had 2.83.[11]

But these reforms—and they have penetrated every aspect of hospital operations—mean that the patients who remain in acute-care facilities are, on average, much sicker than before. The "walking wounded" have been sent home with painkillers and a roll of bandages and left to care for themselves. A good friend of mine in British Columbia went into the hospital at 9:00 in the morning for breast cancer surgery, left for home in the afternoon at 5:00, and had to manage a drainage tube with no assistance or guidance. And these "reforms" were not confined to Canada. Some shocking revelations have been reported in Britain. Alexandra Hospital in Redditch apologized to the families of 38 patients after it was found one patient starved to death, an elderly female patient went unwashed for 11 weeks, some patients died screaming in pain, and nurses taunted their patients.[12] At St. George's Hospital in Tooting, a young patient died of dehydration after phoning police to beg for a drink.[13]

In effect, as hospitals have been forced to become leaner, they have also become meaner. The impact on both patients and nurses is apparent. There is also the growing phenomenon of patient violence toward their caregivers. I doubt this is an unconnected trend. As nurses become more harried, their demeanor may harden. But patients, who are on the receiving end, may push back with resentment. In short, the case for keeping patient care in the hands of humans is weakened if they cannot readily deal with the strains imposed on them. Here, then, is a limited argument for robot caregivers. They don't lose their tempers, they don't become surly, and they don't need sick days.

I think it's reasonable to imagine robots being assigned some of the auxiliary services that support patient care, such as laundry cleaning, instrument sterilization, and, conceivably, food preparation (after all, how could hospital meals cooked by robots be any worse than the present alternative?). And yes, this would cost some employees their jobs. But if we return to the point made earlier—that hospital patients today are, on average, more seriously ill—then it seems to me the case for large-scale robotization falls away. These are patients who are afraid for the future, who are often in great discomfort, and, with the aging of the population, frequently without loved ones in close proximity. The need for human contact and consolation, always one of the duties of nursing, is more important than ever. It would be a serious, indeed inhumane, decision to hand these responsibilities over to machines, no matter how cleverly they are programmed.

I want to turn lastly to distance education. This phenomenon is being heralded as a means of making university classes available to those who could not afford the sky-high fees charged by traditional institutions. And indeed, there is some truth in that. The University of Texas, for example, charges $10,000 for a four-year online course in the humanities. That is far below the price of a comparable degree program taught live on most university campuses. The question is, at what cost? One of the central missions of a university is to stimulate debate, exchange of ideas, and direct exposure to professors who are experts in their field. It might be argued that teleconferencing and webinars in some way offer such experiences. But they are a pale version of the real thing.

Of course, not every professor is a skilled communicator or interrogator. It was said of Isaac Newton, who was required by his Cambridge college to teach at least one lesson a week, that frequently he spoke to an empty room, his lectures being largely unintelligible.[14] Nevertheless, how many students can forget the elevating (though at the time perhaps intimidating) experience of arguing a point of fact or logic with someone far smarter than themselves? Distance education severs this critical link in the development of a young mind. And it does worse. The British Columbia Institute of Technology, for example, offers online courses in nursing, including high-acuity nursing.[15] Likewise, several American postsecondary facilities offer the degree of nurse practitioner online.[16] How this kind of training can be completed through only limited contact with human beings, whether teachers or patients, is beyond me.

Then again, coursework for such classes must, of necessity, be dumbed down and routinized when computer grading is used. Much of the nuance and deeper implications of any field of study are either lost in this process or, at a minimum, diminished. This isn't education; it's education light. Now it must be admitted that many private universities in the United States have brought this on themselves by charging scandalously high tuition fees. When it comes to designing solutions to the threat posed by robotization, the presence of private facilities complicates matters. In Canada, where most universities are public institutions, government regulation is an option. How private schools in the United States are to be led in a different direction is a more difficult matter.

These, then, are some of the destructive effects of increased robotization. The question is what, if anything, should be done. And here it may be helpful, initially, to consider the measures used to minimize the harmful impacts of the first industrial revolution. For I will go on to argue that similar methods can be employed to limit the damage that robotization may impose. As is well known, the first industrial revolution was so greedy for human capital that children were drafted into the workplace. This was not entirely an innovation. Children had worked in the fields alongside their parents as far back as records extend. Indeed, when I was a young boy growing up in Scotland during the 1950s, teenagers were still being given two weeks' vacation during the school year to go and harvest potatoes. But while farm work can be nasty, cold, and dirty, it was never dehumanizing or exploitive. Coal mines and factories are another matter entirely. Uncounted youngsters lost their lives in mine cave-ins caused by methane explosions. They also began the grim process of developing pneumoconiosis through the inhalation of coal dust, an ailment that, in later life, would kill or disable them. Young boys used as chimney sweeps developed testicular cancer as young as nine years of age, through exposure to soot as they wriggled up the insides of smokestacks. Nothing need be said about those dark, satanic mills, except to note that children were accorded no special care or protection from unshielded machinery.

But adult lives, too, were lost as industrialization gathered steam. In the early going, there was scant (if any) regulation of worksites in Europe or North America. Owners set more value on their plants than they did on workers' lives. The latter were expendable; the former was not. Britain took a baby step toward safety enhancement with the introduction of the Health and Morals of Apprentices Act in 1802. Nominally this statute required factories to provide proper ventilation and clean work spaces. But in practice, it was routinely ignored and rarely enforced. Subsequently, in 1847, the British parliament passed a Ten Hours Bill, which limited the hours of work for children to 10 hours a day: Not exactly an enlightened piece of legislation, but it was indicative of prevailing social attitudes. Not until the early 20th century did workplace safety regulations begin taking the shape we know today.

The point I want to draw attention to here is that, left to themselves, employers during the early years of the first industrial revolution showed little care or concern for workplace safety or the exploitation of children. It was left to governments to impose proper safety provisions in the form of increasingly tight restrictions. It was also found necessary to create public agencies like occupational health and safety boards to enforce compliance with worksite regulations. And the creation of these safety regimes took time—half a century or more. Public attitudes change slowly, though arguably faster today than in earlier times.

Here, then, is my presumption: If robotization represents a threat to human employment and to other human relationships, then we cannot expect industry to police itself. Companies are profit seekers; they have no other purpose. If limits are to be placed on the pace and extent of robotization, that task must fall to government. But how is this to be done? Let's start at the broadest level—the workplace as a whole. One obvious difficulty is that any corporation that set limits on the installation of intelligent machinery would quickly lose ground to other firms in the field that had no such scruples. If robotization of patient care became a widespread practice, any private hospital that refused this option would go bankrupt. Equally, any country that adopted job-saving legislation might expect to see a flight of companies to offshore locations with less stringent regulations.

There is a parallel here to the use of performance-enhancing drugs by athletes. Prior to the adoption of drug testing by various international sports bodies, such as the International Olympic Committee, drug doping was common. And this created a dilemma for athletes who may have wanted no part of it, but who realized that if they did not use drugs, the odds of their being competitive were long. The likelihood was that their competitors were using drugs and thereby gaining a near insuperable advantage. It took the introduction of organized drug testing to give athletes the confidence required to avoid this behavior.

An initiative of the same sort will be required to counter the spread of job-killing robots. As with the effort to stop doping, the international community as a whole will have to mobilize. The Organization for Economic Cooperation and Development might present one such venue. Even so, the movement must start somewhere. It will take the leadership of individual member countries to put this issue on the table. And that isn't going to happen until society becomes more conscious of the threat posed by robotization and demands that its politicians implement job-saving measures. This might look like mission impossible. Will it really be feasible to convince, or require, corporations to give up the considerable savings that artificial intelligence offers? Would any government or group of governments take on such a formidable task? All we can say is that governments did act to regulate the workplace during the first industrial revolution, and at least as much is at stake here—namely, the preservation of human employment.

What of health care and distance education? In Canada there is, in principle, a simple solution. Most health care and postsecondary institutions are publicly funded and governed by boards, the majority of whose members are government appointees. Hence, if a public policy decision were taken that robotization of patient care or large-scale use of distance education should be discouraged or sharply limited, the means exist to enforce that policy. The position in the United States is much more complex, with private ownership of these facilities more common. Yet even here, the federal government has, on several occasions, published guidelines covering such matters as affirmative action in university admission policies, Title IX protection against sexual discrimination or harassment on postsecondary campuses, and the Patient Protection and Affordable Care Act, which significantly affected the health insurance industry. If these measures were both politically and constitutionally possible, I can see no reason why similar guidelines could not be adopted limiting robotization in these sectors.

As to what should, or could, be done to deal with the advance of sex robots, I simply have no clue.

From all of these considerations, I draw the following conclusion. Robots, artificial intelligence and smart machines are rapidly expanding their sophistication and reach. Between 2010 and 2018, computing speed increased from just a few hundred calculations per second per dollar, to five billion.[17] The sheer pace of this phenomenon is itself a concern, because whatever threats it embodies may be upon us before we can react. This is, in every sense, a clear and present danger, and yet we appear to be, at the broader societal level, either ignorant of the danger or alarmingly complacent. It falls to each of us to issue a wake-up call. There is a parallel here in the fight to gain voting rights for women. The suffragette movement succeeded because it mobilized public opinion is support of a proposition that could not be morally denied. Equally, the right to work is a claim that, if made with sufficient energy, will surely generate a sympathetic response.

But the time for action is now. For the enemy is not at the gate. He, she, or it lives among us and grows ever more humanlike in form by the day.

Notes

1. James Manyika, Michael Chui, Anu Madgavkar, and Susan Lund, *AI, Automation and the Future of Work*, online "Briefing Note," McKinsey Global Institute, June 18, 2018.

2. Sean Ross, "How Can Industrialization Affect the Economy of Less Developed Countries?" *Investopedia*, www.investopedia.com.

3. Anthony H. Winefield Bob Montgomery, Una Gault, Juanita Muller, John O'gorman, Joseph Reser, and Donald Roland, "The Psychology of Work and Unemployment in Australia Today," *Australian Psychologist*, February 2, 2011.

4. T. Kieselbach and P.G. Svensson, "Health and Social Policy Responses to Unemployment in Europe," *Journal of Social Issues* 44 (1988): 173–91.

5. Emily Aoki, "In Sexless Japan, Almost Half of Single Young Men and Women Are Virgins: Survey," *Japan Times*, September 16, 2016.

6. "Silicone Squeeze: Japanese Men Choose Life with Sex Dolls over Real Women," *Sputnik News*, July 4, 2017.

7. Matthew Griffin, "Artificial Intelligence Diagnoses Disease by Listening to Your Voice," *Fanatical Futurist*, February 17, 2017.

8. David B. Samadi, "Robotic Oncology: Da Vinci Robotic Prostatectomy—A Modern Surgery Choice!" Online summary of Dr. Samadi's work published by Lenox Hill Hospital, New York, NY.

9. Emily Matchar, "A Robot One Day May Draw Your Blood," www.Smithso nian.com, July 13, 2018. Smithsonian.com is an online magazine published by the Smithsonian Institute, Washington, D.C.

10. Paulo Mauro, Rafael Romeu, Ariel Binder, and Asad Zaman, "A Modern History of Fiscal Prudence and Profligacy" (IMF Working Paper No. 13/5, 2013).

11. "List of Countries by Hospital Beds," Wikipedia.com, online article.

12. Laura Donnelly and Josie Ensor, "Victims of Neglect at the Alexandra Hospital," *Telegraph*, December 22, 2012.

13. Telegraph Reporters, "Man, 22, Who Died from Dehydration in Hospital Rang Police for a Drink of Water," *Telegraph*, July 2, 2012.

14. Michael White, *The Last Sorcerer* (New York: Harper Collins, 2012).

15. Specialty Nursing Programs, British Columbia Institute of Technology: School of Health Sciences, online curriculum listing.

16. Online Degrees: Nursepractitionersonline.com

17. Hod Lipson, "Why Most of Us Fail to Grasp Coming Exponential Gains in AI," *Singularity Hub*, July 15, 2018.

CHAPTER TWO

On Passing as Human and Robot Love

Babette Babich

This chapter raises the questions of robot consciousness and the notion of "passing" as a human being. It also considers the related issues and nuances connected to sex robots and our very human willingness to suspend critical thinking in matters romantic, including some crucial limitations of robots as erotic partners.

Turing Tests

Toasters might well "pass" a Turing test, a test named for its originator, Alan Turing, who called it the "imitation game." Turing, a mathematician and code breaker, proposed this test as an ideal for computer or artificial intelligence whereby a questioner would be unable to detect any difference between human responses and machine responses.[1] "Passing" as human is accordingly the ultimate achievement, and the idea of the Turing Test is that users be persuaded that the machine in question has enough signs of intelligence to indicate that some consciousness is behind it.[2]

This is a version of our tendency to attribute nonconsciousness to fantasy beings, such as zombies. Think of the wildly popular AMC television series *The Walking Dead* (2010 and still ongoing as of this writing). It gives rise to a case of what today's analytic philosophy calls the "hard problem of consciousness" (are zombies unconscious? How do we know this?) and what older versions of philosophy called the problem of "other minds" (do other people have minds?). Think of Descartes's example of heavily cloaked human beings who might really be automata. How do we know? In the case of toasters, we may attribute a kind of agency to the machine, blame it for undertoasting or burning our toast, with seemingly no setting in between, as if this were done *purposively*. In the same way, we can hit the wheel of a car that won't start or curse copy machines or printers on the blink just when one needs them most. If an ATM keeps our card, we may be inclined to assume some intent behind the card slot.

Cognitive coherence, or consistency of understanding, turns on semiotic ambiguity, determining the meaning of statements that could have two or more meanings. You ask me—*How are you?* I hear that as only a form of greeting and respond—*How are you?* I haven't answered your question, but it's your turn, *and* because we are talking about you, you don't mind. This is important when it comes to machine consciousness because, as most AI designers realize, if the focus is on ourselves, we pretty much take the machine to mean what we think it is saying.

Transhumanism: On Passing as Human

Sex robots—also sometimes listed under an older patented name, "teledildonics"[3]—can include variations on sexting, sometimes including animatronic strap-ons. More commonly the focus is sex with robots, that is, mostly men having sex with mostly female-looking sex robots, sometimes helpfully described in science fiction as "gynoids," programmed to talk and pitched as a turn-on—which it is, as even a cell phone can have an erotic charge: metonymy works that way.

The Turing test is about faking an exchange such that a machine "passes" as human. Robot sex is a similar deal, and we are set up for this because in the erotic domain, we have long assumed that the only thing that matters is appearance. Remember Nietzsche's nasty comments on women? He calls them "little dressed up lies" in his series of "signposts" to the "great stupidity" that he took himself to exemplify. Nietzsche points at the same time to the efficacy of such deceptions, seducing one's neighbor into a good opinion—and afterward believing piously in just this opinion—and wondering if "a well dressed woman"—being "hardly dressed at all—ever caught a cold"?[4]

Today we are inclined to argue that women dress in such a fashion to please themselves, an odd claim on the face of it; and in *The Second Sex,*

Simone de Beauvoir argued that this is bad faith—well in advance of the current #metoo movement or, indeed, its backlash. Although I do not think de Beauvoir is wrong about the issue of bad faith, a great part of male privilege is the option of not having to have such bad faith.[5]

Fooling other people about one's looks online extends to both women and men, and such bad faith is easy. We call it "curating" and urge that one learn to do it, all the better to market oneself.[6]

Picking a flattering photo for job applications is important, and it is still more important for Internet dating apps. This selectivity generates one the biggest complaints concerning deception on dating sites. Photoshop is everywhere, and, like the stars, we need to control our online image, just as we also want Botox and cosmetic surgery and so on.

And there is no gender divide here. Stuart Heritage, writing for *The Guardian* in a joke essay on the uselessness of Fitbit, points to his own photo: "See that picture of me in the byline? I currently look like I killed and ate that person, then hid from the police by sleeping in a bin for a month."[7] In academia, we sign up for coaches to help tweak résumés and CVs. Some hire experts to design their personal web pages or Facebook presence, Twitter, and so on, and academic counselors almost universally recommend that students look to such advisors, if only as a necessary precaution.

Note that whatever one's position on post-truth, fake news on Tinder or any other dating app is not news—or truth. Such self-representation via Photoshop or simply selecting a more flattering photo (as you get older any photo *younger* than you currently are will do) is the fastest way to the transhumanist strategy. Thus one becomes a ghost surfer on the Internet of lies.

Robo-Sex for Fun and Profit

Who needs a real person with all their real differences from your needs? What do we need people for? Wouldn't a robot be better when it comes to a relationship? We already use robots when we hand an iPad or a cell phone to a toddler: it shuts them up. And then there are applications for the aged and infirm, thinking of jobs no one wants. In conversation, the sociologist and philosopher, Steve Fuller, author of *Humanity 2.0*, pointed out that human caretakers can be cruel, steal, get tired, have bad days, and are rude in almost any case.[8] Why not have a robot care for Grandma or Grandpa, able to shower them with infinite attention, offer infinite patience for their slowness, their deafness, their forgetfulness? Add sex and Viagra, and what more can you ask for? *Ex Machina*–type stories would throw a wrench in that, and thus Hollywood doesn't typically tell such stories (though Ray Bradbury and other science fiction writers have long since explored this terrain). Hollywood overall keeps it light, like *Robot and Frank* or, on the funky dystopian side, *Ghost in the Shell*.

It is a tiny detail that none of our robots are ambulatory, yet our self-absorption and tendency to project onto others rather than listen to them makes conversation with AI-outfitted sex robots seem sufficiently like fascinating conversation. Here, it matters too that some men may be looking for just that level of discourse, quite in the spirit of the line from an old Billy Joel song, *Just the Way You Are*:

> I don't want clever conversation
> I don't want to work that hard

But no matter whether the *level* of conversation might or might not be adequate, it is key to emphasize that sex robots don't move much, and they are typically cold; it's hard to have body-temperature regulation, as it turns out—and, once again, they do not walk, and they do not caress. To be sure, if we did have robots that could walk, there'd be a whole market for amputees and other prosthetic users who could well see the bodies of such robots functioning in applications far more useful than sex.

As for economics, Bill Gates thinks that with robots—provided we tax manufacturers who use them—one can free humans up for the kind of jobs it turns out that robots can't do all that well, such as taking care of the elderly.[9] As Gates put it, "What the world wants is to take this opportunity to make all the goods and services we have today, and free up labor, let us do a better job of reaching out to the elderly, having smaller class sizes, helping kids with special needs." Notice that all the jobs people would thusly be freed up to do are service industry jobs with relatively low pay, such as helping the elderly and teaching special-needs students.

But, Steve Fuller argues, should we not assume that robots would handle such tasks better than we? And what would we care that these, our robot caretakers and educators, are not human? After all, this is the robot fantasy of Asimov's *I, Robot*. Perhaps better for exploring these connections might be the super soldier or supercop long on the military drawing board: not the cyborg hero of *Robo-Cop*, dead but with human elements, but—and much rather—his all-machine, clunky robot adversary. Not surprisingly, when it comes to man versus machine, John Henry style, the man wins, but only in literary fancy. Today, the new remake of

Lost in Space features a nifty new robot, *Iron Man* style. But it is not a bulky machine, we assume. It is a humanoid that drives the future we envision: our ultimate fantasy (think *Blade Runner*) according to Günther Anders and his reflections on what he called our "promethean shame" in his 1956 book, *The Antiquatedness of Humanity*.

The *Robocop* reference, humanoid aesthetics aside, is probably to the point in this age of drones. To go back to what is euphemistically called love, namely, intercourse machines as opposed to killing machines, the allure of the catfish phenomenon is its one-sided malleability. Thus non-reciprocity is the key to the way digital media already works, not just between us and our machines but also with one another, on social media. Our online friends are there for us just and only when we are interested, to the extent we are interested.

In a related fashion, what it means to be attractive to others is to be bodily optimized, cultured to the tastes of the other, and in our culture, that is the male. So we have very little information on the ideal male for a woman, because what women want is for men to want them. The details can be figured out postproduction.

In practice, when it comes to AI as such, this is important for Apple's Siri app and Amazon's Alexa, which have a lot of the features of an ideal girlfriend: the voice sounds young, sounds pretty (think Scarlett Johannsson in *Her*), but most crucial of all, *friendly, positive, no complexity, no troublesome depths or details*. I'd say this is what every prostitute pretends to be as a matter of business practice, and this same superficiality makes it easy to pretend to be someone you are not.

The ideal of a perfect body and of a perfect friend or companion is a streamlined notion that takes negativity for granted. It is a strategy for dealing with trade-offs down the line. One seeks to maximize improvement, so one pays a visit to the hairdresser or the dentist, or for cosmetic Botox; one seeks to improve on a nature one views as needing improvement. This embarrassment concerning what we are by mere nature is the very point of what Günther Anders named our "promethean shame."

Here, think of an ideal fantasy of a sex robot, which one can see in film and on television, oddly enough, often darkly, *Ghost in the Shell* style, or *Black Mirror*. Because our depiction of robots begins on film, if not in print with Mary Shelley's *Frankenstein*, it is worth noting the role of film in depicting or representing robots that are taken to be human. In 1927, Fritz Lang built such sexed robots into his *Metropolis* not by building robots (they were not then, as they are not now, ready for "prime time") but by casting the same actor who played Maria, the subversive organizer and social agitator, to play the robot who was substituted after the agitator in the film story was supposedly killed—a substitute who looked like the original Maria because, of course, the same actor played the robot.

We use human beings to play robots on stage and screen. The actor thus "passes" as a robot as in *HUMⱯNS*, the British television series. Earlier versions of passing as a robot passing as a human being, in addition to the Maria robot, include *Star Trek*'s Data and the human(oid) Seven of Nine and also Jude Law in Steven Spielberg's 2001 *A.I. Artificial Intelligence*.[10]

Jude Law's beauty facilitates our sense of him as a machine. Robots on the screen are thus *not* like the original *Lost in Space* robot but rather the same as a human being, *Westworld* style, *Blade Runner* style. This sameness is utterly different from the sex robots one can buy today at whatever price point.[11] Even the best, at the high end of hype, are easily and obviously distinguishable from human beings. What these "robots" are is upgrades on existing sex dolls, a very profitable industry that turns very much on the fact that, like any sex toy, sex dolls can't be returned for a refund if the toy in question does not look (or feel or work) the way the buyer imagined it might.

Arguments are often made that robots could solve or ameliorate some thorny questions, providing sexual intimacy for the handicapped or—and here it gets thornier still, as we might remember that full-size sex robots tend to be surprisingly small, such that one need change very little for a sex robot to have the features of a preadolescent boy or girl. Yet, experts argue that sex robots can provide helpful outlets for those with questionable sexual proclivities. The ethical problems with this assertion are considerable, and the *HUMⱯNS* series made what was, in effect, a rape of an android the key to the story of consciousness. It is AI, the same key that the same consciousness also turned out to be in the character of the high-end sex robot played by Alicia Vikander in the 2015 film, *Ex Machina*. It seems to be the case that one cannot just do whatever one pleases with a sex robot.[12]

Unboxing the Future of Robot Sex

Current debates regarding sex with robots show what's at stake. To quote the headline of a mid-September 2015 article in the UK newspaper, *Telegraph*: "By 2050, human-on-robot sex will be more common than human-on-human sex, says report."[13] Yet, if the porn industry attests to anything, this commonality is already the case if we can define a robot as a porn site, but we dream of more.

Intriguingly, such sex robots will be, like today's current sex dolls, female-for-male (or male-for-male), rather than male robots specifically designed for female users. In fact, some authors do discuss this, but it is important to foreground the shortcomings of these male robots: none is particularly tall, and they do not move on their own: they are not automata. Indeed, the user of such sex robots seems to do more than a certain amount of heavy lifting, as Karley Sciortino, who tested one such male sex robot, reports: "It's like having sex with a lazy person: You have to do all the moving."[14]

Sense and Sensibility: The Robots We Have versus the Robots We (Might) Desire

The Turing test attests to our desire to be able to avoid being fooled; this, Nietzsche argues, really drives our preference for truth and our anxiety contra the lie—or fake news these days. Hence the holy grail of artificial intelligence: designing a spy code or computer program (or an android) capable of "passing" as a human. The film fantasy ideal of robot love brings in sex, ergo porn. The language of teledildonics gives us sex at a distance.

Let's go back to *Metropolis*—or better still, let's go back to the bio- or soft robots in *Blade Runner*. The iron maiden vision of creating a robot, using sex as a lure to the death, to suppress the yearning for freedom of the worker underclass, is the theme of Fritz Lang's 1927 *Metropolis*. Improve that vision by hacking animal life, and biotech "hacks"—or, better said, hijacks—animal life, and what could be better? With Philip K. Dick's 1968 sci-fi novel *Do Androids Dream of Electric Sheep?*[15] made for the screen as Ridley Scott's 1982 *Blade Runner*, sex with robots became part of the challenge of thinking artificial intelligence, and the recent *Blade Runner 2049* suggests the ultimate biohack: reproduction.

In our teletronic imaginary, sex with a robot would be sex with a perfect replica of a human being, perfect in all ways, especially amiability. The idea further offers something like the *Westworld* fantasy: maybe sex with Anthony Hopkins or, better, Jude Law or, better still, Alexander Skarsgård or Timothy Olyphant; or for a female star object, imagine Carrie Fisher, restored to Princess Leia days forever, or Marilyn Monroe or Brigit Bardot, just to name clichés.

We assume the robot would be just like a human being. And we dream on: imagining them as companions without the negatives of human lovers. Robot lovers wouldn't quarrel with us. Further, they would always be eager to share the same activities *while* evoking, just like the latest iPhone, the envy of friends and strangers: the ultimate electronic accessory.

Sex with robots would also mean never having to say you're sorry to your partner or involve unpleasant encounters with the law (or so one can argue). With robot lovers, no desires would be taboo; everything would be permitted—a great boon for the pedophiles of the world, ditto rape, ditto snuff sex (back to *Westworld* again).

Here there are ethical questions. Why should it be ideal to have a robot, or a synthetic human being, mirror one's desire, do what one wants, anything at all? Just this questionable ideal is a selling point; the sex robot, as noted above, is presented as a prosthesis for the lonely, and everyone (at the right price point), it is promised, might be able thus to have a perfect lover. Prostitution or the escort industry or, in some circles, the match-making industry already promises that. But where the prostitute is paid to behave as a perfectly responsive lover, the lure of robot sex is that consciousness and its unspoken reserves would be eliminated: only *your* desires would matter; the electronic personal companion would exist solely for your pleasure. There would be no cheating; your transhuman companion app would be programmable to your specs, without any pesky interiority to rear up, unwelcome, from some unexpected depth in the robot's psyche. Never mind the *Ex Machina* subplot or *Blade Runner*: the appeal of robot lovers will be their utter slavishness, indistinguishable from human beings; they will be nothing like human beings. This is the heart of the plot, and also the reasons for the name, of *HUMVNS*. And *HUMVNS* raises the uncomfortable question of consciousness—the question of what a complete replica of a human, should it be utterly complete, might entail.

Until we reach that ideal reduplication of the human, sex robots as we have them and imagine them are not presented as passing for human, as such, to any literal extent, but given that they can *seem* to talk, AI-outfitted sex robots are simply better versions of sex dolls already on the market. Some proud owners of these sex robots detach the detachable vaginas from the mechanical lady and wander around with these—so much more portable and more hygienic to boot.[16]

It is already clear that there is a question here. Is there a gender division when it comes to sex robots? Yes, and this is one of the reasons the sex-robot market caters to men. At the same time—and this is more obvious than Donna Haraway's *Simans, Cyborgs, and Women*—were anyone to invent a perfectly proportioned Adonis model that can talk . . . but perhaps even better versions, like a sex robot that would be able to walk and carry things, including perhaps its companion, from time to time . . . think of the romantic appeal of Alan Rickman's Colonel Brandon carrying a nearly drowned Kate Winslet up a hillside to safety in *Emma*

Thompson's screenplay adaptation of *Sense and Sensibility*—and to do so on command, and for as long as one wished to be carried. But also, while we are at it, imagine a nonlazy version of a sex robot, able to make love for hours—the sky would be the limit.

Indeed, once (if) the technical hitches are resolved (I say *if* because these are more complicated than many suppose), one can imagine that in the future, people will arguably prefer robot sex companions and robot lovers to "real" people. If we can have a lover perfectly attuned to our every desire and one that might also help around the house and provide personal transport options, would that not be lovely?

The problem, to go back to the toaster capable of passing a Turing test, to the extent that we attribute purposiveness or intent to it, is capitalism. To this we must add the hype that is probably the most characteristic quality of AI robotics at every level, from sex toys to manufacturing bots and certainly when it comes to replacement limbs or high-tech prosthetics. But—and this is why all of this works—people are amazingly tolerant, amazingly tractable wishful thinkers, which is perhaps why the Turing test works as a test in the first place. Because of this optimism and tolerance, people are prepared to buy items that *do not do* what they are hyped to do and to buy them anyway, because one seemingly *wants* technology to be whatever it claims or promises to be. Hence, although these products are nowhere near beta stage, sex robots are already on the market. Indeed, sex robots have already been ordered, used, and subsequently stashed in closets or sitting motionless on couches.

Notes

1. See Alan M. Turing, "Computing Machinery and Intelligence," *Mind* 49 (1950): 433–60.

2. See instructively, if generically, on this, Tor Norretranders, *The User Illusion: Cutting Consciousness Down to Size* (London: Penguin Press, 1999).

3. See, for history and discussion, Cyrus Farivar, "Cybersex Toy Industry Heats Up as Infamous 'Teledildonics' Patent Climaxes," *Ars Technica*, August 2018.

4. I discuss these and other aphorisms in Babich, "Reading Lou's von Salome's Triangles," *New Nietzsche Studies* 8, nos. 3 and 4 (Winter 2011/Spring 2012): 95–132; as well as Babich, "Nietzsche and Eros between the Devil and God's Deep Blue Sea: The Erotic Valence of Art and the Artist as Actor—Jew—Woman," *Continental Philosophy Review* 33 (2000): 159–88.

5. Babich, "Great Men, Little Black Dresses, & the Virtues of Keeping One's Feet on the Ground," *MP: An Online Feminist Journal* 3, no. 1 (August 2010): 57–78.

6. See, for a start, David Berry, *Critical Theory and the Digital* (London: Bloomsberry, 2015).

7. Stuart Heritage, "Forget Walking 10,000 Steps a Day—I Have Another Solution: Fitness Trackers Are Pointless, Especially When You're Only Walking to the Kitchen for Another Bacon Sandwich," *Guardian*, February 21, 2017.

8. Steve Fuller in Conversation with Babette Babich. *Vimeo*, https://vimeo .com/112417612

9. David Z. Morris, "Bill Gates Says Robots Should Be Taxed Like Workers," *Fortune*, February 18, 2017.

10. I discuss this in Babich, "Friedrich Nietzsche and the Posthuman/ Transhuman in Film and Television," in Michael Hauskeller, Thomas D. Philbeck, and Curtis D. Carbonell, eds., *Palgrave Handbook of Posthumanism in Film and Television* (London: Palgrave/Macmillan, 2015), pp. 45–53.

11. The entire sex robot debate turns on our expectation that technology for full-body replacement is somehow imminent. Theorists contend that the only thing blocking these enhancements are restrictions, ethical (mostly) or financial. But this conviction overlooks technical obstacles.

12. See David J. Gunkel's new book *Robot Rights* (Cambridge: The MIT Press, 2018). These are complex questions and to explore them, see too, quite to the point of the present chapter, Kate Devlin, *Turned On: Science, Sex and Robots* (London: Bloomsbury, 2018) in addition to the contributions of John Danaher, ed., *Robot Sex: Social and Ethical Implications* (Cambridge: The MIT Press, 2017).

13. See Helena Horton, "By 2050, Human-on-Robot Sex Will Be More Common Than Human-on-Human Sex, Says Report," *Telegraph*, September 29, 2015. The article cites the entrepreneurial research report proposed by "futurologist" Ian Pearson, published via the Bondara website for the Internet or mail-order sex shop, a kind of Amazon for porn and porn supplies, "The Rise of the Robosexuals." Intriguingly, such sex robots will be, like today's current sex dolls, female-for-male (or male-for-male) more likely than not. Yet the image on the cover of the literally "pink" graphics paper features a porn-styled, eroticized sketch of a human gal with a male, not at all erotically styled robot—discreetly covered everywhere it matters.

14. See Allison P. Davis, "Are We Ready for Robot Sex? What You Learn about Human Desire When You Get Intimate with a Piece of Talking Silicone," *The Cut*, May 2018, https://www.thecut.com/2018/05/sex-robots-realbotix.html.

15. Philip K. Dick, *Do Androids Dream of Electric Sheep?* (New York: Doubleday, 1968).

16. See, again, Davis, "Are We Ready for Robot Sex?"

CHAPTER THREE

Who Is Responsible for a Self-Driving Car?

Chris Beeman

For a short period of time in the spring of 2018, several news reports surfaced with versions of the following: *Self-driving car kills pedestrian,* and later, *Who is responsible?* Details were initially sketchy. The person killed was a 49-year-old female with a bicycle. Her death occurred in darkness. News reports retrieved online noted that the pedestrian who was killed was homeless.[1] A video clip depicting the incident was soon released, purportedly showing how difficult it would have been for any driver to avoid killing the pedestrian. Soon thereafter, the story left the news cycle. As the story lost prominence, more deeply concerning questions of who bore responsibility, both in ethical and legal senses, for the death of this woman also faded. While earlier concerns about the issue of responsibility in self-driving cars had been raised—when, for example, the testing of a Tesla led to the death of its driver[2]—this was the first publicly announced incident of a self-driving car killing a pedestrian in the United States. Deeper and more concerning questions have gone to the background of a news cycle that hungers only for novelty, yet the incident continues to raise the theoretical and practical question of who is responsible for self-driving cars. More broadly, the question can be asked of any new technology that involves apparently autonomous decision making in a physical world: Who bears responsibility when a human-designed tool or being with some degree of ability to learn, and thus to exceed the original design, acts destructively? The issue of agency is key here because the being in question has something like it, in the sense that it is programmed to respond to circumstances and must "choose" among available options, although its original designer was human. This raises the question: To what extent does an original designer bear responsibility for the unpredictable learning of a nonhuman being? Another question with deeper implications lurks in the background: Can we legitimately refer to machines with a kind of agency (in the sense that they are able to learn, and thus to exceed the imagined parameters of response originally devised by humans) as beings? And how do we treat the actions and choices of these *beings* in an ethical sphere?

I want to set aside, for the time being, a couple of points. The first, applicable in this case and many others to do with new technologies, is that vested interests trump truth. By this I mean that any organization with a vested interest, from private corporations to elected governments, will almost always use arguments for far loftier goals than those actually motivating the adoption of new technologies. While the limitations of space preclude a detailed exploration of this aspect of this story, the effect of this proclivity is made more extreme in the current context in which news feeds available to each citizen widely vary, with algorithmic choices determined by their ability to hook attention rather than to be accurate or truthful.[3] Broadly, the purpose behind the development of driverless vehicles is likely not global happiness or well-being, or mobility for elder drivers, or safer streets, but an intention to make profit. Ready to hand in this case is the oft-repeated justification that these cars will make driving safer for everyone. Viewed this way, from the perspective of financial investors, the threat posed by the killing of a pedestrian is a serious one, albeit an economic rather than an ethical one. Thus, to understand the actions taken afterward, an economic lens is needed. If an ethical lens is used, the actions taken appear deeply lacking. That the arguments being made for the adoption of robotic vehicles are mostly ethical in nature— mobility, public safety, removal of repetitive work from a human sphere, and so on—hardly matters.

Second, I will set aside for the time being (but will come back to later) the way the story of the killing of a pedestrian has been told and what this says about the complicity of corporate media, and thus the shaping of the story. I am thinking in particular of how the effect of this story on major Internet news players such as Facebook, Amazon, and Google, who strongly influence news today, and whose businesses might be benefited by self-driving vehicles, might be viewed. These corporations provide platforms for the distribution of news, including news that affects them. The story noted above has strong implications for these corporations, because it is intimately linked with their own plans for expansion. This is because self-driving vehicles will permit moving seamlessly between virtual and actual worlds, through the distribution channels and delivery vehicles that make possible the physical delivery of virtual desire. By eliminating the need for human deliverers, costs will be cut dramatically. Thus, there would be a natural inclination for news cycles to favor the benefits of driverless technology over the detriments. However, the key question here, that of responsibility, needs to be addressed first.

Responsibility

It must be recalled that the conversation around responsibility regarding self-driving cars began with the killing of a pedestrian. Some claimed that the vehicle could have avoided the person. That is not the point. The point is that, in blunt terms, an algorithm *decided* to kill a person, in the sense that it took decisions leading to the death of the pedestrian.[4] What used to be an excuse for manslaughter with a vehicle—drunkenness—has long been understood to be simply another form of absence of requisite ability for driving. The algorithm was designed by a team of humans; the car and algorithm were made by a corporation; another corporation testing the car wants to use this technology to make money. Yet where does the responsibility lie? No one on the design team can be held responsible: the incident was unforeseeable, we will be told. The human "driver" cannot, because he or she was only monitoring the car. And while the car manufacturer may be held legally responsible, as a corporate entity, and despite its consideration of being a person under the law, it is incapable of an ethical sense or feeling of responsibility. Its duty ends at the fiduciary aspect of things, and this responsibility is a financial one, to its shareholders. Thus, as noted above, the death of a pedestrian from a self-driving vehicle can only be viewed, corporately, as an event with potential financial implications.

The upshot is that there is no*where* to assign responsibility. In this context, I am speaking of responsibility, not legal liability (though that also appears moot). And within *responsibility* I am interested in particular, not only whether a person could be *held* responsible, but whether he or she would *feel* responsible. What prompts me to do so is this: in an imagined future, in which collisions between autonomous vehicles and pedestrians that involve injury to pedestrians increases, it is possible to imagine a scenario in which the human "operator" was never held responsible and learned not to *feel* so. Nowadays, few people would feel responsible if the bus they were traveling on injured a pedestrian. If, in the future, they could *feel* innocent for trusting a system that was intended to be safe but was not—to pedestrians or perhaps to people in vehicles other than their own—then we have an ethical problem: a person would be injured through the actions, direct and indirect, of other people, and no one would feel any responsibility for this. The design team is far too removed from the incident, and the corporation has no capacity for ethical feeling, and the driver has learned to deny any feeling of responsibility. Part of the damage that the killing of this pedestrian and many others in the future may cause is the dehumanizing of people as we learn not to feel responsible for actions of which we form an intimate part.

Even the terms used are laden with import. By using the term "driverless vehicle," one perhaps plays into the hands of car manufacturers, in whose interest it would be to make a seamless transition to this new technology. It is in their interests to make it seem as though nothing really new or big is happening: "just another kind of vehicle, folks." A driverless vehicle is just another wave—which is connected to the ocean of transportation—but which happens to one be of the future. Subsequently, I wonder, what are the people in the vehicle called? Certainly, some are passengers. But all wouldn't be; would anyone be capable of "driving" a driverless vehicle?

I think car manufacturers will want there to be someone "in the driver's seat" as this transition occurs, someone to whom responsibility can seem to temporarily fall, even though these "drivers" will quickly learn, in synchrony with their trust in the technology, not to feel responsible. And it is not that they will actually be paying attention. I have to wonder what, exactly, was the person employed to be sitting in the vehicle monitoring the test doing at the time of the collision? It is unlikely he or she will be held responsible and may not feel so. The act of driving is distinctly different from that of being a passenger. How were these individuals able to move between the roles of being attentive and of determining the passage of the car, to one of allowing the car to take over, and back again?

To avoid confusion, we should perhaps speak not of "driverless vehicle" and "operator" but of operator and robot. No, not even that works: if the vehicle is really robotic, then there is no immediate human controller. Thus, given the information available on the technology now, it appears there is a robot that is carrying passengers, at least one of whom will be nominally called a driver. So, let me use the terms *robotic vehicle* and *ostensive driver* to apply to them.

To explore this further, I want to suggest a thought experiment that will shed light on what an ethically oriented person—the kind we want to be "driving"—and who is the ostensive driver in robotic vehicle at a time that it strikes and injures a pedestrian, might feel. What ought an ethically oriented person to feel in such a circumstance?

To begin to answer this, I am going to invoke a story told long ago by an acquaintance about driving in a country in the Middle East, in a time of conflict. The story goes that she had arranged for a taxi. The driver drove dangerously fast, as they always did there in those times. On a couple of occasions, she requested that the driver slow down but never demanded it. In a busy area, she saw a child starting to cross the road just ahead of the vehicle. There was a loud thump. She looked back to see what had happened. She couldn't see the child. She asked the driver to stop, but he did not. In the local culture, this kind of incident was viewed as regrettable but understandable collateral damage in getting from one place to another. This event had happened many years before I heard of it. Yet my acquaintance still had thoughts about it, wondered if the child had been hit, wondered if he or she had been seriously injured or perhaps killed. There was no way to trace the incident—she didn't even know the area well enough to find the location where it had occurred, but she somehow felt some responsibility for what had happened.

If I read the signals of my acquaintance's expression correctly, she was feeling remorse, as if she were in some sense responsible. All kinds of factors might have mitigated against this feeling: the culture and its style of driving, pedestrians' understanding of this, the fact that she had made some slight attempts to slow the driver, the uncertainty over what had actually occurred, the fact that this occurred in a circumstance of conflict during which the speed her vehicle was traveling at reduced danger to her and the driver. And yet, even many years later, she felt some responsibility for a possible incident that only *might* have happened.

I mention this story because it might hint as to how an ethically oriented person might respond in a circumstance in which a vehicle that carries her, and which in some sense she bears responsibility—although not for its direct control—causes harm. If this is the way in which humans would or perhaps should feel, then such feelings ought to be part of the way in which robotic vehicles are programmed. This would mean that, among other things, the remorse felt by my acquaintance, or "felt" by an operating system, could change future driving behavior, and perhaps do so ineluctably. It is beside the point that at present, it would not be possible for a machine to feel this way; such feelings, despite their complexity, that would be completely comprehensible to most sensible adults, ought to be at the heart of ethical decision making. And they ought to be at the heart of designing algorithms that control driving. Despite this, while machines can learn, they cannot ethically learn through, among other things, the feeling of certain emotions. I want to suggest that being in a certain emotional state might be requisite for learning certain ethical principles. And if it is understood that almost all actions have ethical import—not just the obvious cases of vehicles moving at high speed risking lives—then we are at an impasse when it comes to trying to include ethics in programming. And if we cannot, we have to admit we are willfully adopting technologies that will transgress ethical boundaries.

I would posit that the position of being in the taxi, above, might feel different to the bus example raised earlier for several reasons. The first is that the taxi is only moving in a public space because a particular party requested it. A bus just runs on a particular route, so an individual's own responsibility for it being there is lessened, though not nil: by being a passenger, one contributes to the perceived need for a bus to be traveling that route. But in the case of the taxi, there is greater responsibility for a vehicle being in that particular place and time because the passenger has requested it (though one might suggest that the request was made with the tacit understanding that it be *safely* there). There is also the intimacy of a car and the physical proximity of a pedestrian being struck that is different from the relative anonymity due to physical distance on a bus. One more thing occurs to me in noting this story: that there was some component of personal safety for my acquaintance and her taxi driver driving in ways that might be unsafe to others. By moving faster, they became a more difficult target to hit, as it were. Thus, her driver might have been intentionally putting these concerns above concerns for others who were not employing him, or to which he felt a lessened degree of responsibility.

Surely, this last point is relevant in regulating the design of algorithms that relate to robotic vehicles. If they favor the safety of those in the vehicle, then this, by necessity, compromises the safety of all other citizens. Decisions will be programmed that make "choices" between safety of the passengers in the vehicle and those in other vehicles, or who are not in vehicles. Who—I hope it is a human—will choose between these choices? What ethical parameters will programs be developed under? And who will monitor the choices made? Will there be illicit or "black market" sales of algorithms that will be distinctly dangerous to others and will favor the passengers' safety?[5]

But perhaps it is more nefarious than this. Perhaps what is most protected will not be the pedestrian or the passenger but rather the corporation manufacturing the technology, with robotic vehicles comprising a new category of "citizen." There would be an inherent interest on the part of that corporation, in case it could be held responsible, to have the kind of accident that left no trace that could bring legal liability, and if there were a trace, it would be reduced to the minimum payments for injury. As a truck driver I happened to get a ride with while hitchhiking once said to me, he had been instructed, if a collision were unavoidable, to "make it good." A dead person was less costly to the company that employed him than a disabled one.

Emotion and Responsibility

The Middle East taxi story above could provide some assistance in making sense of what it might be to make an ethical decision at all. In the circumstance of moving through a public space, presumably, from the case given, it would mean a process of gradually becoming better and better at discerning the interface between one's interests and use of space and those of others And this would be done through experiencing feelings and working through how one might act in response to these negative and positive feelings, with emotional imagination for others' states of being in order to act—and feel—in the world more ethically.

This is thus a very contextual way of moving through the world. Yet the at the heart of creating algorithms is designing set "responses" in advance, that is, of necessity, at some distance removed from the very circumstances that might promote or give the necessary context for ethical learning. In designing algorithms, judgments have to be made in advance. This means that while attempts may be made to incorporate context, the actual context of this particular decision as it occurs in real time will not be taken into account. This is because a decision has been made according to certain principles, prior to this moment. Is a baby's life worth more than an older person's? What if it is *your* baby? And when it comes to it, are we humans comfortable in a system that requires the determining of actions based on principles alone? Don't we want, sometimes, to be acting in perhaps ethically uncertain ways, but in ways that every person—or parent—would understand and probably agree with? Without feelings, it would be impossible to program a machine to be able to do this.

News That Controls the Story

Of course, the ways the corporate news media have addressed this story puts into question neutrality in coverage. For example, a recently accessed online story[6] begins with the title, "Uber Mishap Raises

Questions: Who's Responsible if a Self-Driving Car Breaks the Law?" An initial reasonable question is why the killing of a pedestrian is referred to as a "mishap" if not to diminish the event's apparent importance. The word also makes the story seem as though there was a technical problem. But there has been no evidence released yet to show that the problem was technical; it is entirely possible that the algorithms governing the operation of the vehicle were operating perfectly and that the death of the pedestrian was due to these, rather than despite these. The story continues, "The investigation into the Uber crash that killed a Valley homeless woman is still in its early stages." While it could be argued that this is simply reporting style, to give human context, the victim's social status is likely to influence public opinion against her. It is possible that the victim's being homeless would put into question her legitimacy or capacity as a pedestrian. The report continues, "But preliminary reports from Tempe police show the victim, Elaine Herzberg, 49, was jaywalking when the self-driving car hit her on. . . ." Why is her jaywalking of significance? Is it because jaywalking is unsafe and illegal in some areas? Is it meant to excuse the inability of a robotic vehicle to sense the presence of a pedestrian?

The questions about such corporate reporting could go on, but the limitations of space permit me to mention only a few further troubling questions that emerge from reporting around the incident. First, who released—and on whose authority—the video images? Were these changed in any way? What say did the dead person or those close to her have over the release of the image of her dying? Why is the public screening of this death different than the troubling graphic depictions of executions? What might be the interests of corporate media and manufacturers and users of robotic vehicles in releasing these images?

Then, the awkwardly constructed news story suddenly turns back to interview Attorney James Arrowood, who says, "The good news out of this particular tragedy is we will have more information than we have ever had in an auto accident." Perhaps the sense given in the article, that this is not really a tragedy at all but an opportunity for new knowledge, is due to the awkwardness of the writing style, so let me leave it for the time being. Let me leave also the likelihood that the beneficiaries of this knowledge—"the good news"—will be the manufacturers of robotic vehicles, who may use the knowledge to create even safer vehicles, rather than pedestrians. The underlying premise of this article appears to be much more troubling than its all-too-familiar, cavalier attitude toward the victim: the premise appears to be that with more information about an auto accident, purely technological problems to do with writing better software will be solved. Thus, the way the story has been told, it has become technologized: it is about a car that malfunctioned and will, with the integration of information coming from this regrettable mishap, operate better in the future, rather than about the death of a pedestrian, of a life that will not be lived.

But the problem is not lack of information; we already are aware of the apparently increased ability of robotic cars to accumulate more information that pertains to avoiding a collision. The problem is what to do with it absent a body and feelings. The premise I would like to introduce here and continue in the next section is that, without a body, what constitutes an ethical action cannot be fully understood and enacted. Because a robot is not a human being, and yet is being asked to act like a human being, this might be a fatal argument for the capacity for nonhuman beings to act in the physical world in circumstances with ethical import.

The particularly damning aspect of this argument for robotic vehicles, if it holds, is that if there is no body (constituting or containing or communicating with mind and emotion), then it will be known in advance there could have been no ethical decision taken. This will not prevent unethical acts from being committed by nonhuman beings. Quite the opposite—if they are done, they will have been consciously condoned, with the knowledge that they are not ethical. Thus, if legislated, an apparently unavoidable conclusion would be that the underlying constructs of at least some of the constituencies of the global, modern West are intentionally absent of ethical consideration—something of which even we, and even in this particular phase of human history, are unlikely to willingly approve.

The Importance of Body for Ethical Decision Making and Responsibility

As it normally does, *The Guardian* gave more compassionate and balanced coverage to this story. In a March 19, 2018, article by Sam Levin and Julia Carrie Wong,[7] John M. Simpson, a privacy and technology project director with Consumer Watchdog, is quoted as saying, "The robot cars cannot accurately predict human behavior, and the real problem comes in the interaction between humans and robot vehicles. . . ." I imagine a human driver seeing a cyclist walking with a bike and perhaps some groceries, and this driver might, perhaps unconsciously, *feel* what it is like to be in that position. I have been in the position many times of having to carry groceries home by bike. Say the groceries are suspended on the handlebars in a plastic shopping bag because they are heavy to carry. The bag sways slightly with each step, and the overall motion of the bike is made wobbly by the changing forces of each step. In the same way I have just done, a driver present in this case might, as it were, put him- or herself in the position of the other, the person walking a little unsteadily because the grocery bag is unsteady. This might be just for a moment, possibly quite unconsciously. The driver might imagine him- or herself having some challenges to walking confidently in this context. And as this occurs, the foot of a skilled driver will be raised from the accelerator pedal and will be poised above the brake in anticipation of having to slow suddenly. This latter step involves connecting what is perhaps an unconscious feeling to the action of driving, and not all drivers will act in this way. But the point I wish to emphasize is that it is initiated by the feeling of compassion for or understanding of another person, and this is rooted in the perception, at a probably unconscious level, of sameness in position. The driver feels something that a machine cannot, because he or she has a body that registers sensations that would equate with walking, with a bicycle, with a swaying shopping bag.

And the technician hearing this, who (odds against) feels the necessity of humanity in the equation, might think, "Okay. Good point. Shopping bag. Bicycle. We have image recognition technology. We'll put those in right away."[8] And of course, this will completely miss the point. The point is that for the deciding algorithm to correctly respond to the circumstance, it would need to have a body (that feels) to which it could unconsciously refer in an entirely unpredicted and unknown in advance way in order for it to act ethically. It would need to be able to check a circumstance against its own (vulnerable) well-being, in an imagined future case.

Perhaps it might be replied that a body, per se, might not be required, but only the accurate imagination of one. This argument relies on the word *accurate*. In this case, I believe for accuracy to be attained, the imagined body would have to give signals in all ways that a real (human) body would, in order for ethical decision making to occur. So, we are back to a kind of Turing test,[9] although in this case, it is a more challenging one. In this case, the robot would have to be able to imagine itself with the vulnerability of a human body, within the realm of variation of most human bodies, accurately enough that it could posit its own body in similar position to the bodies it registers through its sensing devices. The probable impossibility of this is akin to, though perhaps more damning than, the argument made above about the necessity of feeling certain feelings being at the heart of ethical decision making. In both cases, a machine without these would not have the capacity to invoke these human aspects in making decisions with human interests in mind.

But even supposing some kind of advanced artificial intelligence were developed and could be put into practice, there would still be a problem. It is that ethical decision making would have to be given over completely to a machine. For a human operator to try to be involved would only muddle the equation and perhaps, as above, in crucial milliseconds, cause error. Thus, there would have to be sufficient confidence in an algorithm designed to make decisions in advance, confidence that it could respond the way a human would in cases such as the one noted at the heart of this paper. This, in turn, takes decision making out of the realm of the ethical because, as already noted, ethical decisions, to qualify as I am defining them, have to be not only made from within a human physical body, with concomitant emotions, but also responding to real circumstances and must not be simply running an algorithm, which cannot, by definition, be adequately tuned to the particular moment of the ethical decision. The particular distinction about ethical decisions in driving circumstances is that they happen in milliseconds. Humans don't resolutely compare utilitarian, pragmatist, and idealist interpretations of an event in order to determine which might apply; they feel and act. If a machine does not do this, then it is simply running a program rather than acting ethically. If this does not occur, we will have made lawful a machine doing potentially life-threatening things in public with no ethical supervision.

Lessons from Prince Edward Island

The abbreviated version of what will transpire in the future with robotic vehicles is that these cars will be adopted, except in some poor countries and in some very progressive ones. They are too potentially profitable to not be. The misleading argument—that they are safer than human drivers—misses the point: no one can be held responsible for them. And because we live in a world of cars, and these will be seen as an improvement on cars, we cannot imagine a world without them. We will come to think of them as being necessary, and we have forgotten that only a few generations ago, cars were not even around, and that only a few places actively approved them at their inception. In most places, with the intentional dismantling of public transportation systems, they just became the norm.

A little over a hundred years ago, in Canada's littlest province, Prince Edward Island (PEI), cars were banned.[10] The irony for the current discussion in this chapter is that, at the time, they were referred to as *horseless carriages*. So, at that time, the debate was over not whether humans should be part of the equation of transportation, but whether horses should. And this could easily be used to ridicule current arguments of the kind I am making. Such a tack misses the point here, which is that, in both the case of horse-driven and horseless carriages, human ethical judgment and responsibility is needed.

As it turns out, PEI was also the province with the first automobiles in Canada—in fact from 1866, in what was then called British North America—just before Canada was created. Yet, in 1907, about 40 years after their inception, they were banned from public roads.[11] The simple fact is that they proved to be a nuisance to people, and the predominant form of transportation and work, the horse, was disturbed and frightened by them. Rather than let the situation get out of control, a ban was issued, which lasted about five years. Only when external pressure overruled local sentiment were cars permitted. The idea that a living being, and not even a human one, could be given precedence over a nonliving instrument seems almost like a fairy tale in its quaintness to us nowadays.

But the instrument changed the whole game. Ultimately, after a time of pause, the feelings of horses were addressed by killing them or letting them die off, thus not having any horse feelings to worry about. Economic systems have never been kind. But they have, at least until now, had identifiable human proponents. The interests of car manufacturers were quite evident at the turn of the last century. One way to understand the issue of robotic vehicles is to look for which corporations will most benefit from them.

The main point of the story of PEI is not to give some quaint example of an obviously erroneous superannuated view but rather to note that, at a certain point in the past, cars were not the norm. At some point, people in PEI consciously chose to overturn the interests of horses and many people in favor of economic advance. Using the misleading argument of roads being shared spaces, cars forced animals, most public transportation, and pedestrians off them. The fact that it is an island (now, alas, connected by a thoroughfare) is of significance here. By virtue of a physical boundary, this was one of the few places where the new normal of automobiles did not just simply expand into available space. The dark side of cars—their violence, their use as weapons, the dangerous mingling with intoxicants, their noise, the deaths resulting from not just collisions but the necessary emissions of poisons—arguments that were raised at the time on PEI and are now ridiculed[12]—all have been overlooked or forgotten. It is seen as quaint to challenge the car at all.

Afterthoughts: Is AI SF?

It is likely that, from a future place with robotic cars, the decision we face now over their fate, *at the time that a decision can still be taken*, will be seen as hopelessly naive. But it is not just that robotic cars will, due to economic pressure, overturn the need for ethical decision making. If the argument above holds, then the known and predictable inability of a robotic vehicle to make the ethical decisions will have been intentionally chosen by some of the beings who do have the ability to ethically decide. This would be more ironic were it not so tragic. In the same way horseless carriages took over roads by using the argument that roads were shared public places, while ignoring the asymmetrical effect cars would have on animals, human drivers will also be quickly eliminated. In the example from PEI, a relatively loud engine, which is part of what makes a car go, scares a horse, the horse bolts and thus becomes unsafe. What about when a robotic vehicle does what is safe for it, but not for a regular driver? Say the robotic vehicle is following at a safe distance for its capacity to react, but that the distance is not safe for human drivers, and it is perceived as being unsafe by human drivers. There may be initial laws stipulating against this, but there will be irresistible pressure to go as fast as is possible, even if humans perceive this as being unsafe. The lesson from PEI is clear: when cars became popular, horses became the minority. Once in the minority, there was no longer room to hold concern over the feelings or safety of horses—or other humans; they were now in the minority. If a robotic vehicle doesn't "intend" to threaten a crash, but acts in ways that are safe for it but that feel unsafe to a human driver, would this kind of action truly permit human drivers to continue driving? It is likely that humans will stop driving because it will be impossible to tell whether such actions are performed by a human driver behaving recklessly, with too little tolerance for error, or a robotic vehicle, driving with narrower tolerance than the humans around it know they themselves would need. As one's driving style influences that of others, this will likely have a domino effect on human-controlled driving as well. Ultimately, this will lead to humans being forced not to drive, in the same way horses were forced off PEI roads.

The truly chilling idea of where responsibility would lie, in a more distant future, if AI were attained in vehicle design, is that it would fall to the car itself. It would come about thus. The designers would have provided algorithms capable of learning. The parallel might be to a safe driving instructor giving sound instruction. But ultimately, responsibility would fall to the controlling force of the vehicle to drive safely. When there is no driver, but there is AI or something like the capacity to make choices, it must fall to the controlling agent with the intelligence. It cannot fall to the instructor or algorithm designer. And it would be of no use to try to hold the manufacturing company responsible; once it leaves the factory, a vehicle with AI must be assumed to be acting on its own. And of course, this scenario would occur well past the time when an ostensive human driver would be required to sit "in the driving seat." Thus, forgetting even ethical responsibility of the kind addressed above, the only player who could be held legally liable in a truly robotic car employing AI would be the vehicle itself. And with this comes the concern that although legal responsibility could be applied to the vehicle, the very felt sense of responsibility, which is dependent upon a body and the emotions that I alluded to earlier, would be utterly lacking. This is due to an inability to position oneself as a human, viscerally, affectively, and ethically, whose welfare ought to be considered. This means that a lack of emotional capability, and the lack of a body to hold those emotions, would be impediments to the very kind of learning that would be required for the touted prospective of greater safety (for people) to occur.

In other words, we know that an earlier supplanting of horsepower with the car shifted the meaning of human movement, from one whose pace was allied to the pace and sensibility of animals to something much more alienating and individualistic. Robotic vehicles will again reshape movement, and again in ways that could not have been imagined at the point in time when the majority had not yet made the shift—namely, while change was still in the control of people. The proposed shift willingly takes on the possibility of movement, normally to be considered a basic right, controlled by principles and forces that we know to be incapable of ethical decision making, as interpreted above. Thus, the probable future of movement looks bleak, indeed.

Notes

1. Angie Kohler, "Uber Mishap Raises Questions: Who Is Responsible if a Self-Driving Car Breaks the Law?" *ABC15 News*, March 20, 2018, https://www.abc15.com/news/let-joe-know/uber-mishap-raises-questions-whos-responsible-when-an-unmanned-car-breaks-the-law.

2. "Tesla Car That Crashed and Killed Driver Was Running on Autopilot, Firm Says," *Guardian*, March 31, 2018, https://www.theguardian.com/technology/2018/mar/31/tesla-car-crash-autopilot-mountain-view.

3. Canadian Broadcasting Corporation, *Sunday Edition*, September 1, 2018, https://www.cbc.ca/radio/thesundayedition. Vis also a chapter by the author in this volume.

4. As this chapter is going to press, I note an article printed after the initial story of a collision causing the death of a pedestrian in *The Information* (May 7, 2018), confirming the suggestions made herein. It reports, "The car's sensors

detected the pedestrian, who was crossing the street with a bicycle, but Uber's software decided it didn't need to react right away. That's a result of how the software is tuned. Like other autonomous vehicle systems, Uber's software has the ability to ignore 'false positives,' or *objects in its path that wouldn't actually be a problem for the vehicle* [my emphasis] such as a plastic bag floating over the road. In this case, Uber executives believe the company's system was tuned so that it reacted less to such objects . . . the tuning went too far, and the car didn't react fast enough." Accessed at https://www.theinformation.com/articles/uber-finds -deadly-accident-likely-caused-by-software-set-to-ignore-objects-on-road.

5. Ibid.

6. *ABC15 News*, op cit.

7. Sam Levin and Julia Carrie Wong, *Guardian Weekly*, March 19, 2018, https://www.theguardian.com/technology/2018/mar/19/uber-self-driving-car-kills-woman-arizona-tempe.

8. See footnote 7.

9. Wikipedia (accessed October, 2018) defines the Turing test as "a test of a machine's ability to exhibit intelligent behavior equivalent to, or indistinguishable from, that of a human. Alan Turing proposed this in 1950." Accessed at https://en.wikipedia.org/wiki/Turing_test.

10. Greg Williams, "When P.E.I. was the Last Holdout Against the Motorcar," *Driving.ca*, August 22, 2017, https://driving.ca/auto-news/news/horse-power-ru led-p-e-i-in-the-early-19th-century.

11. Ibid.

12. Ibid.

CHAPTER FOUR

Who's Your Mama? Assisted Reproductive Technology and the Meaning of Motherhood

Jennifer Parks

Assisted reproductive technology (ART) allows infertile people to have biologically related children, but it is changing what it means to be a mother. Previously a mother was the person whose egg and gestational labor produced a child, and she was also the one who engaged in the social activity of raising that child. The notion of "mothering" has not included gay couples, as it has always been assumed that only women can mother. But now that more same-sex couples are seeking out assisted reproduction for family-making, we need to rethink who counts as mother and what mothering labor entails. Does donating an egg make one a mother? Does serving as a gestational surrogate constitute mothering? Could same-sex couples be mothers? The woman who intends to be the social parent intends to be the mother but plays no part at the point of birth—is she a mother? All of this leads to philosophical, legal, and moral confusion, worsened by different players contesting their roles and laying claim to the identity of mother. This chapter considers the challenge

ART poses to a traditional understanding of motherhood. Appealing to philosopher Sara Ruddick's notion of "mothering persons" and "maternal practice," the essay will argue for a more inclusive understanding that does not limit mothering to women alone.

Introduction

Reproduction is leaving the bedroom and moving to the laboratory. While certainly most children are still conceived and gestated the old-fashioned way, with the advent of assisted reproductive technology (ART), an increasing number of children come into the world using some kind of reproductive assistance. This is certainly not a new occurrence, given the availability of ART for the past 40 years: after all, the first IVF baby, Louise Brown, was born in 1978, and services have expanded quickly since then. Recent decades in particular have seen an unprecedented number of techniques and applications come into practice such that practitioners are laboring within what has been called "the wild west of reproductive medicine,"[1] where few rules apply and what is possible outstrips concerns for whether we ought to be doing it.

This essay concerns ART as enabling technology and considers its effects on how we understand who is—and what it means to be—a mother. While the role and definition of "mother" might seem universal, unchanging, and eternal, the degree to which the advent of ART has complicated it is noteworthy. In particular, what counts as maternal work, and even who counts as mother, is now contested and uncertain.[2]

Are You My Mother?

Consider the beloved 1960 children's book, *Are You My Mother?* by P. D. Eastman.[3] That book follows a baby bird as he hatches and then searches for his missing mother while she is out in search of food for her hatchling. Along the way, he encounters a variety of other creatures, including a kitten, a hen, a dog, and objects like a boat, an airplane, and a bulldozer, asking them all the eponymous question ("Are you my mother?"). The story and illustrations appeal to some quite questionable normative tropes of its time, with the mother bird identified and gendered by depicting her wearing a scarf, and the suggestion that, when it comes to mothers and their children, "like belongs with like." (When he finally gets returned to the nest, and his mother asks him, "Do you know who I am?" the baby bird states, "Yes, I know who you are. . . You are not a kitten. You are not a hen. You are not a dog. You are not a cow. You are not a boat, or a plane, or a Snort. You are a bird and you are my mother!")

This was my favorite book as a child, and with good reason. The story depicts the comfort and certainty of knowing who your mother is and that she loves you unconditionally. The final illustration depicts the baby bird under the protective wing of the mama bird, who feeds and protects him. The book presents the ideals of "good" mothering in its appeal to traditional conceptions of "mother."[4]

Fast forward almost 60 years since that book first appeared, and the theme and title take on all new meaning. The question, "Are you my mother?" seemingly so easily answered decades ago, is now more uncertain. With the advent of ART, and its corresponding disintegration of biological, gestational, and social motherhood, it is unclear who now counts as mother—or, perhaps more importantly from a child's point of view, who can be counted on as mother. Before proceeding with these concerns, however, I will consider the various ARTs that are currently in use and those that promise to be widely available in the future.

The State of the ART

The term "assisted reproductive technology" (ART) refers to any reproductive intervention or technique that involves the external handling and/or manipulation of human gametes such that fertilization and development occur outside the human body. ART includes a variety of techniques and interventions; below I briefly highlight some of the more popular techniques to provide a general overview of what the practices entail.

In vitro fertilization (IVF): Many heterosexual couples diagnosed with infertility turn to IVF services to achieve a pregnancy using their own eggs and sperm. In such cases a woman will take fertility drugs to stimulate hyperovulation such that she produces multiple eggs in a cycle. Once the oocytes develop, she undergoes retrieval in a clinic using guided laparoscopy. The collected eggs are fertilized with her partner's sperm (obtained in the clinic via sperm donation) in a petri dish, and they begin the division process in vitro. The embryos are shortly thereafter returned to the woman's uterus in the hopes that implantation will occur.[5] Gay couples also use IVF to achieve at least partial biological parenthood: one partner's sperm is introduced in vitro to eggs harvested from a donor they select. The fertilized embryos are then implanted in a surrogate for gestation so that, in the end, the gay couple receives the child to raise as their own. Generally, for any couple pursuing IVF, the purpose is to allow at least a partial biological connection to the resulting child(ren), so couples will use their own gametes wherever possible.

Commercial gestational surrogacy: The practice of commercial gestational surrogacy often follows an IVF cycle in cases where the commissioning woman cannot (or does not want to) carry a pregnancy, or where gay couples need a woman to gestate the embryos created through IVF. In cases of commercial gestational surrogacy, the commissioning couple hires a woman (usually via a clinic) to gestate and carry their embryo(s) to term; the surrogate turns over to the commissioning couple the infant that is born so they can serve as the social parents and raise the child. To better secure their parental rights over the children that result, commissioning couples are increasingly likely to seek an egg donor separately so that the commercial surrogate is not the biological mother.[6] There is now a robust global market in reproductive travel and tourism, where couples from wealthy countries travel to less developed nations to find inexpensive services, including surrogacy services. The global practice is also driven by a lack of services available in couples' home countries, necessitating that they go abroad to seek these services elsewhere.[7]

Gamete donation: As noted above, heterosexual couples who commission IVF services prefer to use their own gametes to create embryos, cementing their full biological connection to any children that result. In cases where this is not possible, however, they will turn to egg or sperm donation to create embryos, facilitated by third-party providers. And out of necessity, gay couples select egg donors and lesbian couples choose sperm donors as a matter of course in pursuing their reproductive ends. While in many countries the selling of gametes is prohibited, the United States allows a market where egg and sperm "donors" can receive payment (often generous payment)[8] for their gametes. Potential donors undergo a rigorous selection process, which for most clinics results in less than 5 percent being accepted into their egg or sperm donor programs. Commissioning couples (whether gay, lesbian, or heterosexual) choose their gamete donors from websites that feature the donors, which provide photos (sometimes including childhood photos) and information about the donors' educational, familial, and genetic history. Couples choosing gamete donors can thus select donors that best "match" their own characteristics, mimicking as much as possible a biological connection. However, the selection process also allows couples to select for characteristics such as intelligence, athleticism, and beauty, encouraging a market for the most "desirable" characteristics.[9]

Women who are selected to serve as egg donors must undergo the same procedures as noted above in the IVF process; however, instead of having the eggs harvested for their own purposes, they are given to couples who select that donor. As some authors have noted,[10] these young women undergo reproductive risks for the sake of others and sometimes compromise their own fertility when complications such as ovarian hyperstimulation syndrome (OHSS) occurs.[11] Men who are selected as sperm donors follow a simple donation process in clinics, where their sperm is collected by clinicians.

Beyond these popular ART services, there are new, cutting-edge, and highly contested reproductive practices that have been approved for use in humans within some jurisdictions. These services are described below:

- 3-parent IVF: As a way of avoiding the birth of children with mitochondrial DNA disease, a new practice that is referred to in the popular press as "3-parent IVF" has been implemented. This technique involves the IVF services noted above for a couple but adds in a third party—an egg donor whose egg "shell" is used, and into which the biological mother's egg nucleus is inserted. By using the donor woman's egg shell, the transmission of mitochondrial DNA disease is avoided.

    The controversy surrounding this new technique is twofold: first, it concerns the unknown long-term effects of the technique and its potential to pass alterations on to future generations in the family line where it is used with females; and second, it concerns the involvement of three parents, to which some commentators object on moral grounds. Given the miniscule amount of DNA in the donor woman's egg shell, it is not agreed that deeming this technique as "3-parent IVF" is very accurate.[12] This treatment is available in some countries, like England, but is currently banned in other countries (like the United States) until further research is done.

- Ectogenesis: Finally, while not yet perfected, some research labs are working on ectogenesis, or the ability to gestate fetuses outside a woman's uterus. The Children's Hospital of Philadelphia (CHOP) in Pennsylvania has had some success in gestating lamb fetuses in "biobags," thick plastic bag–like substances that are intended to mimic the uterine environment.[13] This technology is proving tricky to perfect, as much is still not known regarding the choreography of gestation and how the maternal body interacts with the fetus during the gestational process. But there is no question that this technology will eventually be perfected and that there will be a market for it. It is being pursued at facilities like CHOP for use with premature infants but could also be used in the future for women who cannot or prefer not to carry pregnancies, or by gay couples who wish to avoid hiring the services of a surrogate. As I will later argue, the use of ectogenesis for these purposes is morally troubling, as it would mean the complete elimination of human beings from the gestation and birthing process, leaving children at even greater risk of being abandoned to the technologies that create them.

ART as Enabling Technology

In the introduction to this essay I noted that the various forms of ART are "enabling" technologies. I refer to ART as enabling technology because it offers individuals and couples the chance to have (biologically related) children when it would otherwise not be possible. In some cases, a couple cannot biologically reproduce without assistance because of infertility experienced by either or both partners in a heterosexual relationship. In other cases, the partners might be involved in a same-sex relationship such that unassisted reproduction is not possible. (A gay couple, for example, need an egg donor and surrogate to reproduce.) In still other situations, one or both partners may not desire or value the experience of pregnancy and gestation, though they desire a child, and so they choose to hire others to provide these services for them. ART enables couples in such situations to try for a child (and even a biologically related or par-tially biologically related child). It enables them to achieve the goal of having children.

What ART does *not* do is offer individuals or couples a "cure" for infer-tility or for their genetic conditions. The techniques available allow indi-viduals to circumvent their infertility, but they do nothing to fix or change it. For example, after an IVF cycle to create embryos for implantation, a woman is just as infertile as she was before it; likewise, "3-parent IVF" does not cure mitochondrial DNA disease. Thus, we cannot speak of ART as treating or curing infertility, but we can speak of it as affording some persons the opportunity to make biologically related children where it would otherwise be impossible.

ART is enabling technology because it allows otherwise childless indi-viduals and couples to achieve the goal of having biologically related chil-dren.[14] But it also enables same-sex and queer couples to form families in a variety of novel ways. Through the advent of ART, we have seen the "queering" of families, where gays, lesbians, and other individuals use various technologies to create families in a variety of formations. ART is thus often praised for breaking the bonds of heterosexual, biological reproduction by extending it to nontraditional families; however, it has also been a Pandora's box in the legal, ethical, and social problems that it has created. Below I consider some recent cases that exemplify how the practice of ART has put at risk the well-being and protection of the children that resulted.

Case 1

In an infamous 2008 case, a Japanese couple contracted an Indian woman to gestate a child, relying on the husband's sperm and donor ova. Before the child was born, the couple divorced. Both the commissioning mother and the surrogate refused responsibility for the child. The husband could not be recognized as the father of the child because India does not permit removal of children by single men. For a time, Baby Manji had not only no legally recognized parent but was also stateless. The child's Japanese grandmother eventually secured custody of her, and India issued her a certificate of identity that was enough documentation to eventually take her to Japan in the care of her grandmother and father.[15]

Case 2

In 2015 an Italian gay couple used surrogacy services in California, where the gestational woman carried a twin pregnancy and gave birth to their boys. Both men used IVF to create genetically related embryos, and the gestational woman used her own eggs, so that the boys have the same mother and were carried in a twin pregnancy. But "when the two men returned to Milan with their newborns, a clerk at the registry office refused to transcribe the babies' birth certificates, barring the men from registering the boys as their legal children."[16] Following the clerk's refusal, the couple petitioned to register as their children's parents; the initial court ruling refused, but upon appeal each man was permitted to register his biological son as his own. While this allowed the men to seek Italian citizenship for each child, "the babies cannot be recognized as children of the couple, nor are they to be considered brothers, even though they share the same genetic mother, who donated both eggs."[17]

Case 3

In May 2014, American actress Sherri Shepherd filed for divorce from her husband, Lamar Sally. Prior to the divorce filing, Shepherd and Sally had entered into a commercial surrogacy contract with a Pennsylvania woman who carried the pregnancy for the couple using Lamar Sally's sperm and donor ova. During divorce proceedings, Shepherd attempted to void the surrogacy contract, refusing responsibility for the baby boy that was being gestated. When the lower court ruled against her attempt to nullify the contract, Shepherd turned to the appeals court in Pennsylvania, which refused to hear her case and required her, as the boy's legal mother, to provide child support payments. Shepherd has not seen the child since his birth and has refused contact with him.[18]

Case 4

Melissa Cook was a 47-year-old California surrogate who made news in 2015 when she went public with her feud with Chester Moore Jr., the biological father who paid her $33,000 to have a child by in vitro fertilization. Moore provided his own sperm and used an egg donor to create the embryos that were implanted in Cook. Citing concerns that Moore would not be able to properly care for the triplets that she birthed, Cook filed a lawsuit to challenge the constitutionality of California's surrogacy law, which treats the intending parents as the only legal parents of surrogate-born children, and which terminates before birth the surrogate's parental rights to the children that result. Her suit was rejected by the court.

In July 2017, Cook appealed her case with the U.S. Supreme Court, where she claimed that the California surrogacy laws violate the Fourteenth Amendment. According to the appeal, "Cook asked the justices to decide six constitutional questions, including whether California's Gestational Surrogacy Statute violates the equal protection or substantive and procedural due process rights of either surrogates or babies born to surrogates."[19] The Supreme Court ultimately refused to hear the appeal, and as a result Chester Moore Jr. remains the only recognized parent to the triplets.

All the cases above included use of IVF, donor egg and/or sperm, and gestational surrogacy. They indicate the complex legal, social, and ethical issues that arise when ART is employed to break down what has historically been the unified roles of genetic, gestational, and social mother, or when it extends family making to gay couples, where no mother may be present at all. In what follows below, I will consider the significance of compartmentalizing these steps in the production of a child, which has increasingly had the unfortunate result of putting the children that result at risk of abandonment.[20]

Who's Your Mama?[21]

Historically, and quite generally speaking, the woman who gave birth to a child was unproblematically the mother. Prior to the availability of assisted reproduction, the biological, gestational, and birthing woman was mostly (though not always because of the possibility of an implant) one and the same; this made it straightforward to determine who was the mother, for legal and social purposes. The challenge children faced within the legal system was in determining paternity (and the associated economic responsibility for a child).

Yet, with the rise of assisted reproduction, it became possible to separate the genetic, gestational, and social aspects of mothering. Egg donors supply the oocytes required for reproduction, but in almost all cases they are not the gestational or social mothers. Surrogates may be hired to carry a pregnancy, but in most contemporary practice, it is not their eggs used to create the embryos. And the woman who commissions the egg donor and surrogate may be neither the genetic nor gestational mother, but she takes on the role of the social mother who raises and cares for the child. This compartmentalization of motherhood has led to difficult questions regarding who is the mother in any given reproductive situation: what does "mothering activity" constitute (e.g., Is it producing the eggs from which the children result? Is it the work as a gestator? Is it being the social mother who is responsible for raising the child? Or could it be all of these?)?

With the *dis*-integration of mothering comes the need to reconsider what mothering entails, and who is a mother. Why does this matter?

1. It matters for legal purposes, because courts must determine in various circumstances which mothering claim has force or, in situations of abandonment, who is legally responsible for a child.

2. It matters for financial reasons, as assignation of motherhood carries with it significant financial responsibility for a child. (Note Sherri Shepherd's refusal to accept responsibility for her surrogate-born son to avoid such financial obligations).

3. It matters for moral reasons, because we need norms in place to secure mothering or maternal practice to ensure children are loved, valued, and reared appropriately.

4. It matters for social purposes, as members of the community need to know who holds the identity of mother and who should be held responsible for a child (as a simple example, school administrators need to know whom to call in cases of emergency).

Currently, however, in ART we lack agreement about and conceptual clarity surrounding the categories of mother and mothering. For example, some commentators on gestational surrogacy reject the surrogate language because they view gestational labor as mothering work.[22] Other commentators explicitly reject any mothering language, choosing distancing terms for these women, like "commercial surrogate," "gestational surrogate," or—most distancing of all—"vessel."[23] Similarly, on some accounts the women who supply their eggs for others to create a child are simply providers of genetic materials, with no mothering status. On other accounts, they are biological mothers who wrongly attempt to separate themselves from the children that result.[24] An increasing number of children born of egg or sperm donorship search for their gamete donors because they feel a deep desire to know their biological roots and to connect to their "real" parents. This highlights the conflict around whether egg donors or gestational women are mothers, engaging in mothering practice in some way, or whether they are mere suppliers of wombs and genetic materials that are not meaningfully connected to mothering activity. These questions will be addressed in more detail in what follows.

Romanticizing Mothers and Motherhood

My particular emphasis on the compartmentalization of motherhood via ART and the problems that result is not meant to hearken back to a romanticized, idealized conception of motherhood. On the contrary, I recognize that mothers have (and historically have had) the ability to be cruel and abusive to children and that some children do not experience mothering as a nurturing and loving connection. Yet one can recognize the evils that can attach to some mothering without dismissing all of it as morally bad. Despite examples of damaging mothering practice, I argue that children nevertheless need a mothering person, someone who is tasked with the special obligation of care that comes with the birth of a completely needy and helpless infant.[25] As Eva Kittay has eloquently stated in her work on dependence and dependency relationships, we are all "some mother's child,"[26] and—I would add—we all ought to have access to that identity as *being* "some mother's child." It is morally wrong to deny any child that identity.

To build on this claim that mothering is essential to children, I appeal to Sara Ruddick's work, *Maternal Thinking*,[27] which attempts to describe the kind of thinking that derives from the work that mothers do. Ruddick's account, almost 30 years old, still resonates in an age of ART because it allows us to consider mothering as attitude, work, and practice. In such a way, we can examine the compartmentalization of mothering activities in ART to help us determine which (if any) of them constitute mothering practice. It is also noteworthy that Ruddick's account does not associate maternal thinking or practice with women alone; on the contrary, her approach allows for and encourages maternal thinking and practice in men. This is especially important in an age of ART where an increasing number of children are born to gay couples and a female is not necessarily part of the family unit.

On Maternal Thinking and Practice

According to Ruddick, maternal work involves preserving, nurturing, and socializing a child so that he or she will be socially accepted.[28] How this is done may vary from culture to culture, but any claim to motherhood would involve at least some aspects of these activities. In keeping with Ruddick's account, I suggest that we need to reject any core or defining essence to motherhood. As Hilde and James Lindemann Nelson have noted in their work on families, "Romanticism and cynicism must be avoided if we are to come to any sensible understanding [of motherhood]. . . . Instead, we can think of [mothers] as people clustered into configurations that have at least some of a wide array of characteristics, no one of which is definitive, but most of which will be present to one degree or another."[29] This "family resemblance" approach to motherhood allows for cultural variability and flexibility in how we understand it, but it also allows us to set out activities that are likely "to be present to one degree or another." It is important to note that in what follows, my comments about mothering come from the perspective of a middle-class, high-tech culture that largely values biological ties and that has traditionally viewed the nuclear, two-parent, heterosexual family unit as the norm.[30]

Ruddick distinguishes gestation and birthing from mothering. She claims that "neither pregnancy nor birth is much like mothering. Mothering is an ongoing organized set of activities that require discipline and active attention. It is best divided among several people who, in an egalitarian society, would be as likely to be male as female. Birthing labor, by contrast, is essentially female, performed by one woman (aided in many ways by others). Pregnant women—especially if they look forward to mothering—often take a maternal attitude toward the fetus, becoming deeply attached to an infant they have yet to meet."[31] She rejects gestation as mothering, because it does not require discipline and active attention; she claims that pregnancy is more about self-care, as the pregnant woman primarily cares for herself, and the fetus only secondarily receives care from that self-care.

At the point of birth, claims Ruddick, mothering is a *prospective* activity, and as such she notes that all mothers are, in some sense, "adoptive."

As she writes: "All mothers are 'adoptive.' Even the most passionately loving birth-giver engages in a social, adoptive act when she commits herself
to sustain an infant in the world. . . . Generally, since no life can survive
without mothering, the defining hope of birth is to create a life-to-be-
mothered."[32] This notion that all mothers are adoptive and that it is prospective work fits well within the parameters of ART, where in many
cases the intentional, commissioning, social mother-to-be has no biological or labor-based mothering claim until the point at which she receives
the child. It also accounts for the fact that some mothering persons will
not be female, allowing for a more robust understanding of mothering.
The notion of all mothers as "adoptive" recognizes that motherhood is
prospective prior to the birth and receipt of a child, as that is when the
"real" work of mothering begins.[33]

Maternal Practice and ART

Ruddick's account of maternal thinking has interesting implications
for assisted reproductive technology. Here I will only consider the *moral*
claim to maternal status and will leave aside legal considerations. Clearly,
the more closely connected a woman is to the biological, gestational, and
social labor of raising a child, the less problematic is her status and identity as "mother." A woman who undergoes in vitro fertilization using her
own eggs, and who has the resulting embryos returned to her uterus for
implantation, can unproblematically make the claim that she is mother to
the resulting child. After all, her efforts and intentions are geared toward
the birth of a child that she will raise herself and for whom she assumes
responsibility. We might consider this a "simple case" of IVF,[34] as the
three separate stages of IVF all involve the same woman and her own
oocytes. In such cases, as Ruddick phrases it, a woman is involved with a
child's "preservation, growth, and social acceptability," which is "consti-
tutive of maternal practice."[35] In such situations, women cannot so easily
abandon a child as was the case with Baby Manji and Baby Shepherd,
because they are intimately involved in the gestation and birth of their
babies.[36]

As additional contributors are involved in a child's production, maternal work gets broken down into component parts, and the risk of abandonment increases. If a person commissions a woman to gestate embryos,
then the question is raised about the maternal status of that gestator: what
might one say if the gestating woman makes a maternal claim over the
child that results? This was the case for Melissa Cook, who claimed a

right to know and raise the triplets, as she spent nine months nurturing and gestating them, even though her eggs were not used to create them.

Ruddick's claims notwithstanding, I argue that gestational women like Cook *do* have standing in relation to the child that results, given the months of labor and care that they put into the development of the individual. Pregnancy is not a passive state but rather, as commentators like Iris Marion Young and Margaret Little[37] have noted, a unique phenomenon that entails a relationship of intimacy between the pregnant woman and the fetus. Any surrogacy contract aside, a woman who commits to such gestational labor is actively engaged in, as Ruddick phrases it, "maintaining conditions of growth." Indeed, commissioning couples expect no less than this when they select a gestational surrogate to carry a fetus (or fetuses) to term. They select women whom they believe will be able to detach emotionally from the child at birth while still having a maternal attitude toward the fetus during the period of gestation. A number of qualitative studies have indicated that gestational surrogates may develop a maternal stance toward the fetuses they gestate and that they may form attachments to the children that result.[38] Thus, I find it problematic to deny the legitimacy of a gestational woman's claim to maternal status over the resulting child, even in cases where she is not the egg donor. Certainly, such a maternal claim, if it occurs, is not the end of the story in terms of who should be granted *legal* responsibility for the child. But I believe that dismissing these moral claims as fictions wrongs the women who do such gestational labor.[39]

Because gestational women are contractually denied any legal standing through their pregnancies, and in fact they are discouraged from bonding by use of "vessel" language, any sense of connection that may develop should not be used as an excuse to allow commissioning couples to back out and abandon the pregnancies they commission. But it might mean that, where women like Cook petition for consideration, their claim should be given credence, and parental rights should be negotiated in family court. Thus, despite Ruddick's claim that "neither pregnancy nor birth is much like mothering," I argue that her account of maternal thinking and maternal practice give us grounds for seeing gestational women as doing maternal work.

Egg donation is a trickier issue. On one hand, the women who serve as egg donors play an integral role in the production of the child that results. Unlike sperm donation, egg donation is a labor intensive, potentially risky process that requires weeks or months of effort to produce the desired eggs. And like the selection of gestational surrogates, egg donors are often chosen based on their demonstrated caring attitude toward the commissioning couples and the possible future children. Egg donors are expected to convey an altruistic motivation for doing the donation, lest their reasons for doing the donation appear mercenary.[40]

However, a major factor is missing that would support the view that egg donation is mothering activity: there is no fetus or even embryo in relationship to which the egg donor can develop maternal attitudes or to which she can contribute maternal labor. Ruddick aptly notes that there can be no mother without a child: "The concept of 'mother' depends on that of 'child,' a creature considered to be a value and in need of protection."[41] In addition to the fact that there is no fetus or child to which the egg donor can stand in relationship, Christine Overall argues that one cannot claim ownership over a child simply because it derives from one's gametes:

> The fact that a man can be considered to own his sperm and a woman can be considered to own her ovum provides no basis for saying that they own the child who grows from their gametes. A person who owns the materials from which something is constructed, even when those materials are necessary to the construction, does not necessarily own the final product. In this case, the final "product," the infant, is much more than and quite different from the original ingredients, the gametes.[42]

Note that the same applies to concerns about "3-parent IVF" as the woman who donates the egg shell is not "mothering" a developing embryo or fetus (indeed, one does not even exist), so it is not mothering work as Ruddick describes it.

To contrast the role played by the egg donor and the gestational woman, note that in the case of the egg donor, fertilization has not even occurred, and it is not certain that her donation will, in fact, result in the creation of any embryos. Yet the gestational woman spends 24 hours a day, 7 days a week nurturing and developing the embryo into a fetus and, ultimately, a born infant. Indeed, at the point of birth, I suggest that none of the other actors who are party to the creation of the resulting child has as strong a maternal claim to it as the gestational woman, despite what the law might dictate. It is she who has spent nine months in intimate connection to the resulting child, and it is her voice and movements to which the fetus has been attuned. By contrast, the woman or man who would raise the child as social parent is essentially a stranger to the child at birth; he or she is the "adoptive" mother to whom Ruddick refers. The gestational woman is *not* a stranger or "adoptive" mother in that sense, I argue, because she has already been engaged in mothering work.

So, what of those who would serve as social mothers, then? As I previously noted, at the point of birth in assisted reproduction, they are not mothers in any biological or physical sense of contributing oocytes or reproductive labor. And, as I also suggested, at birth when children are handed over for social mothers to raise, their moral claims can be seen to be weaker than those of the gestational women. Yet one might see those who commission surrogacy as mothers in their hearts and minds: it is *their* intentions and actions that made the conditions possible for the child's existence. They have not yet performed the mothering work to which gestational women can lay claim, but it is their *intention* to do so. Given these considerations, it makes sense to recognize these prospective mothers as legally responsible for the children who result, as it is their intention to be fully responsible for the difficult work of preserving, nurturing, and socializing them. Yet their mothering grows and develops over time and is solidified in practice and attitude; it does not arrive full-fledged when the child is placed in their arms. Sherri Shepherd may be a legal mother, but she is clearly not *morally* thinking or acting as a mother. The Italian gay couple who petitioned the court for legal rights over their children were not recognized as legal parents, but they were already morally thinking and acting as mothering persons in their earnest desire to love and protect their children.

From these observations one can conclude that no mothering claim is incontestable, and neither should it be if we are to act in children's best interests. We need to avoid conceptions of mothering that treat it as a zero-sum game, with winners and losers. Indeed, there has been some change occurring in cases of open adoption and open surrogacy, where children have knowledge of and relationships with the women who birthed them. This is beneficial in giving them access to more, rather than fewer, mothering persons who care for and about them.

So, I argue that children *need* mothers: that is, persons who have ultimate responsibility for them and who uniquely and intimately know and love them. But this does not have to mean that all other maternal work and mothering claims need to be erased and denied. Mothering persons can recognize the collaborative efforts that went into bringing their children into being; in cases where other persons acted maternally to help bring about a child's existence, those rearing the child should not view and treat it as a threat to acknowledge and celebrate those maternal contributions.[43]

The Future: Children without Mothers?

Consider again the promise of ectogenesis: the gestation of fetuses ex utero, in "biobags" that mimic the uterine environment. Above all other ARTs, this application threatens the mother/child connection and risks leaving children born without any maternal connections whatsoever.[44] On this ground alone, I argue that ectogenesis is morally problematic and is not something that should be pursued without serious investigation into its likely ethical and social/political implications. As I have noted elsewhere,[45] technologies such as IVF, egg donation, and surrogacy already leave some children born of ART in tenuous family situations, and these are situations wherein they at least have gestational connections to real, human women. It is hard to imagine how the lack of human connection to the processes of fertilization, gestation, and birth might impact a sense of responsibility for and connection to the children who result. Given the weakening sense of responsibility that some would-be parents *already* have to the children whose births they commission, one might suspect that it would be even easier to walk away from a child who is created using donor egg and sperm and gestated ex utero, where a couple has no biological or physical connection to the child who will be born. Shepherd is just one example of the lack of moral seriousness with which some individuals removed from the process treat their maternal obligations; one can only imagine the lightheartedness with which people might treat babies who are so far removed from human procreation as to be gestated in "biobags."

Conclusions

Proponents of ART might view the end of motherhood as a victory for both women and nonheteronormative families.[46] By eliminating these categories and instead identifying persons as "parents," we avoid the artificial imposition of old, outdated, heteronormative categories.[47] Ending "motherhood" might also resist the historically sexist and conservative view of women as solely responsible for reproduction and childrearing. But I argue that eliminating mothers is *not* a desirable goal; when understood inclusively, mothering persons are particular individuals who are uniquely responsible for the protection, development, and socializing of their children—an important role indeed.[48]

Yet even as we extend the definition of "mother" and maternal work beyond women, we must not pretend that women have not historically been and are not still uniquely held to gendered expectations of childbearing and rearing. As Ruddick notes, "we cannot at will transcend a gender division of labor that has shaped our minds and lives."[49] While ART is growing and spreading globally as a practice, and it continues to challenge our understanding of "mother" and mothering, the fact is that worldwide, most babies will still be born to women who are biologically, gestationally, and socially their mothers. In such cases, we should strengthen our resolve to ensure that women everywhere have the means to successfully mother children for preservation, growth, and social acceptability. And in cases where ART is employed in ways that compartmentalize maternal activities, we should be clear about what counts as mothering work and who is the mother so that the risk of child abandonment will be minimized. This essay is an attempt to find such clarity to advance the conversation about what mothering activity involves, suggesting that we can expand the definition of "mothering persons" to include gay men who do the vital work of raising their children.

ART is enabling technology, and it has brought about positive changes in reproduction and family making that have allowed for a wider variety of family formations, at the same time making it possible for people to have biological children who might not otherwise be able to do so. But it has also loosened a sense of connection to the children who are born, potentially putting at risk the notion that we are all "some mother's child." This is a notion of which we cannot afford to lose sight. Like the baby bird in Eastman's 1960 book, any child who asks the question, "Are you my mother?" deserves a clear and affirmative response. It is the least, morally speaking, that we owe any child.

Notes

1. This term has been used by a variety of authors. As examples, see Meredith Leigh Birdsall, "An Exploration of The 'Wild West' of Reproductive Technology: Ethical and Feminist Perspectives on Sex-Selection Practices in the United States," *William & Mary Journal of Women and the Law* 17, no. 1 (2010): 224–47; Benjamin Williams, "Screening for Children: Choice and Chance in the 'Wild West' of Reproductive Medicine," *George Washington Law Review* 79, no 4 (2011): 1305–42.

2. This chapter will focus on women's mothering practices because they have been most central to reproduction and reproductive work and because women's roles as mothers are being compartmentalized by assisted reproduction. It is difficult to avoid referring specifically to women when talking about mothering, as most maternal work is still associated with women's bodies. But I will also be addressing gay parents, arguing that gay men can "mother" their

children by way of maternal thinking and practice such that they can be recognized as mothering persons, too.

3. P.D. Eastman, *Are You My Mother?* (New York: Random House Inc., 1960).

4. Obviously, given the time during which this book was published, mothering was associated solely and uniquely with women. Prior to the advent and expansion of assisted reproduction, it was unthinkable that any child could be reared in a family that did not include a woman/mother who gestated, birthed, and raised the child.

5. The number of embryos returned to a woman in this process varies. In some European countries, single embryo transfer (SET) is mandated in younger women, where one embryo is returned. In other countries, like the United States, numerous embryos have been returned, resulting in a high rate of multifetal pregnancies. The most recent recommendation by the American Society for Reproductive Medicine, however, is that no more than one to two embryos be returned in order to avoid the risks associated with high-order multifetal pregnancies. See Practice Committee of the American Society for Reproductive Medicine, "Guidance on the Limits to the Number of Embryos to Transfer: A Committee Opinion," *Fertility and Sterility* 107, no. 4 (2017): 901–3.

6. The egg donation and gestation processes are separated for a variety of reasons, including the motive of weakening any sense of the surrogate's investment in, and connection to, the resulting child. As noted by VIOS Fertility Institute, "The costs associated with a surrogate tend to be lower than a gestational carrier because a separate egg donor isn't needed. However, the emotional/legal risk of using a traditional surrogate greatly outweighs the potential cost savings. Traditional surrogates have been known to change their mind once a child is born. Depending on the laws of the state where the child is born, gestational surrogacy contracts are not enforceable" (https://viosfertility.com/infertility -treatments/third-party-reproduction/gestational-carrier/).

7. Eric Blyth and Abigail Ferrand, "Reproductive Tourism—A Price Worth Paying for Reproductive Autonomy?" *Critical Social Policy* 25, no. 1 (2005): 91–114. Note that many gay couples use global surrogacy services because they are often prohibited domestically from doing so.

8. In 2016 a class-action lawsuit successfully removed the previous recommendations by the American Society of Reproductive Medicine (ASRM) and Society for Assisted Reproductive Technology (SART) that caps be placed on how much women can be paid for egg donation in the United States. See *Lindsay Kamakahi v. American Society for Reproductive Medicine*, class action complaint, case no. 3:11-CV-1781 (N D Cal), filed April 12, 2011.

9. Indeed, "premiere" egg and sperm donors—those who are the most beautiful, educated, athletic—can command much higher prices for their gametes than their less-well-endowed counterparts. While allowing for higher payments based on desired characteristics has in the past been rejected on ethical grounds, a class-action suit (see note 7) has eliminated any proposed limits on fees for egg and sperm donation in the United States.

10. Bonnie Steinbock, "Payment for Egg Donation and Surrogacy," *Mount Sinai Journal of Medicine* 71, no. 4 (2004): 255–65.

11. Ovarian hyperstimulation syndrome (OHSS) is a medical condition that can occur in some women, particularly those who take fertility medication to stimulate egg growth. Although most cases are mild, in rare instances the condition is severe enough to cause serious illness or death.

12. Francoise Baylis, "The Ethics of Creating Children with Three Genetic Parents," *Reproductive Biomedicine Online* 26 (2013): 531–34.

13. http://www.sciencemag.org/news/2017/04/fluid-filled-biobag-allows-premature-lambs-develop-outside-womb.

14. Note that even partial biological connections are desired. For example, in cases where a gay couple commission an egg donor and surrogate, the sperm from one of the men will be used so that at least one partner will be the biological parent to the child; the other man will adopt the child so that he has legal status as parent to the child. For lesbian couples, one partner will use her egg with a sperm donor and the other will legally adopt the child.

15. See P. Sehgal, "Reproductive Tourism Soars in India: Adoption and Surrogacy Laws Have Yet to Catch Up," *WIP*, 2008, http://www.thewip.net/contributors/2008/10/reproductive_tourism_soars_in.html.

16. See A. Momigliano, "These Two Baby Boys Are Twins, but an Italian Court Says They Aren't Brothers," *Washington Post*, https://www.washingtonpost.com/news/worldviews/wp/2017/01/08/these-two-baby-boys-are-twins-but-an-italian-court-says-they-arent-brothers/?utm_term=.e83464867aa1.

17. Ibid.

18. N.H. Sodoma and Nadia A. Margherio, "Surrogacy & Sherri Shepherd: A Troubling Case," *Huffington Post*, 2016, http://www.huffingtonpost.com/nicole-h-sodoma/surrogacy-sherri-shepherd_b_9152642.html. Note that despite the court's finding that Shepherd is the mother to the baby and financially responsible to him, Shepherd did not define herself as his mother. "Mother" is thus also a personal identity that can be rejected by an individual even in the face legal definitions as such.

19. Margot Cleveland, "Supreme Court Refuses Surrogacy Case of Mother Pressured to Abort Triplet," *Federalist*, http://thefederalist.com/2017/10/03/supreme-court-refuses-hear-surrogacy-case-mother-pressured-abort-extra-triplet/.

20. In some of the cases I note here, the babies were abandoned, even if only for a brief period. Defenders of a liberal approach to commercial surrogacy claim that the law can adjudicate cases where maternal rights are claimed (as in Cook's case) or when a child is left parentless (as in Baby Manji's case). According to this argument, babies are legally protected from total abandonment. For moral reasons, however, I argue that we should be concerned about reproductive practices that put children at *risk* of abandonment, even if such abandonment is averted via legal measures.

21. This section specifically addresses women and the complexity of determining motherhood in light of ART, where the steps associated with the

production of a child are completed by different women. In a later section I will address Sara Ruddick's notion that "mothering persons" can include men as well, meaning that gay men can also be mothers.

22. For example, see Christine Overall, "Reproductive 'Surrogacy' and Parental Licensing," *Bioethics* 29, no. 5 (2015): 353–61. As she notes, "A woman who gestates a baby for a commissioning couple or individual is, I assume, a genuine mother. Gestation is a sufficient condition for parenthood."

23. Such language is noted in Timothy Murphy and Jennifer Parks, "So Not Mothers: Responsibility for Surrogate Orphans," *Journal of Medical Ethics* 44, no. 8 (2017): 551–54.

24. On why egg and sperm donation are problematic, see Melissa Moschella, "The Wrongness of Third-Party Assisted Reproduction: A Natural Law Account," *Christian Bioethics* 22, no. 2 (2016): 104–21.

25. Again, this mothering person could be a man, because, as noted below, the account offered by Ruddick encourages the view that mothering activity is not restricted to women and that, in fact, it should be shared equally by women and men.

26. Eva Kittay, *Love's Labor: Essays on Women, Equality, and Dependency* (New York: Routledge, 1999).

27. Sara Ruddick, *Maternal Thinking: Toward a Politics of Peace* (New York: Ballantine Books, 1989).

28. Ibid., p. 22.

29. Hilde L. Nelson and James L. Nelson, *The Patient in the Family: An Ethics of Medicine and Families* (New York: Routledge, 1995), 34–35.

30. We thus need to consider the particular social histories and social norms surrounding mothering and maternal work and note that some mothers in resource-poor countries may require more resources and assistance than mothers in resource rich countries in order to do the work of loving and preserving their children. We also need to account for changes in family making brought about by ART such that we include consideration for GLTBQ family formation.

31. Ruddick, p. 50.

32. Ibid., p. 51.

33. Note again that Ruddick is speaking in moral terms. Legally in many jurisdictions, the person or persons who intend and commission the birth of children in ART are considered the only legal parents, and they are the only persons with legal rights over a child. This is why Melissa Cook was denied any parental rights despite the gestational labor she contributed; Chester Moore intended and commissioned the birth of the babies, so according to the state of California he had sole legal rights over and responsibility for the triplets that were born.

34. Peter Singer, "IVF: The Simple Case," in William B. Weil Jr. and Martin Benjamin, eds., *Ethical Issues at the Outset of Life* (Boston, MA and Oxford: Blackwell Scientific Publications, 1987), 44–49.

35. Ruddick, p. 22.

36. I recognize that any woman can abandon a child—even a woman who is the biological, gestational, and birth mother. But the compartmentalization of these reproductive roles made it much easier and more likely for abandonment to occur in the cases of Manji and Shepherd.

37. See Iris Marion Young, *Throwing Like a Girl: And Other Essays in Feminist Philosophy and Social Theory* (Indianapolis: Indiana University Press, 1990) and Margaret Olivia Little, "Abortion, Intimacy, and the Duty to Gestate," *Ethical Theory and Moral Practice* 2, no. 3 (1999): 295–312.

38. See Amrita Pande, *Wombs in Labor: Transnational Commercial Surrogacy in India* (New York: Columbia University Press, 2014).

39. I hold this view without regard to whether the parents-to-be are a heterosexual or same-sex couple. Although it is understandable that these couples might want to minimize the emotional connection that the gestational woman might develop for her fetus, denying her moral perspective on the pregnancy or her emotional connection robs her of moral agency.

40. K. O'Reilly, "Egged On: The Commodified Altruism of the Assisted-Reproduction Industry," *Bitch Magazine*, 2016, https://bitchmedia.org/article/egged-commodified-altruism-assisted-reproduction-industry.

41. Ruddick, p. 22.

42. Christine Overall, "Reproductive 'Surrogacy' and Parental Licensing," *Bioethics* 29, no. 5 (2015): 355.

43. This applies to cases of adoption as well as assisted reproduction. Denying or even concealing a birth mother's role in bringing a child into being wrongs both that birth mother and the child who results, creating a legacy of deceit surrounding a child's history.

44. Here I am not speaking about the technology applied to premature infants, as they have parents intent on saving them, and their gestation would be transferred from a woman's uterus to a biobag only because of premature birth. I critique here applications where ectogenesis is used to replace rather than assist the gestation and birth of infants.

45. Jennifer Parks, "Care Ethics and the Global Practice of Commercial Surrogacy," *Bioethics* 24, no. 7 (2010): 333–40.

46. See Anna Smajdor, "The Moral Imperative for Ectogenesis," *Cambridge Quarterly of Healthcare Ethics* 16 (2007): 336–45; Shulamith Firestone, *The Dialectic of Sex: The Case for Feminist Revolution* (New York: William Morrow and Company, Inc., 1970); and Darren Rosenblum, "Unsex Mothering: Toward a New Culture of Parenting," *Harvard Journal of Law & Gender* 35, no. 57 (2012), http://digitalcommons.pace.edu/lawfaculty/827/.

47. Note that we could use the term "parent" for legal purposes—for example, to name persons on a child's passport—which would be desirable for a variety of reasons; but we could maintain the use of "mother" and "mothering" for other purposes. Certainly, many women still value the role and identity of mother and would be loath to give it up. And I suspect that men would also value the identity of "mothering person" given its connotation of intimate association with a

child. Rather than expunging "mothering" from our vocabulary, I argue that we should extend it to be more inclusive of current family formations.

48. Critics might claim that this makes nannies, day care workers, grandparents, and other very involved caregivers "mothers," as these are all people whose roles involve the preserving, nurturing, and socializing work that Ruddick discusses. Ruddick's account would certainly recognize such care work as involving maternal thinking (including care work for the elderly, persons with disabilities, etc.). But mothering involves cases where one is held *uniquely* responsible for the preservation and care of a child, and while such caregivers involved in a child's life are, indeed, held to standards of care, they are not those who are uniquely responsible (legally, morally, and socially) and they are not viewed by others as such.

49. Ruddick, p. 41.

CHAPTER FIVE

Screen Autism, Cell Phone Zombies, and GPS Mutes

Babette Babich

Here we examine the increasing threat of surveillance posed by new information technologies, their contribution to fake news, and their impact on the way we orient ourselves in the world around us. By "new information technologies," I mean not just communication devices like cell phones, social media outlets, and the Internet, but also the emergence of omnipresent surveillance systems like airport security scanners and closed-circuit cameras that can observe our every move in public places.

Surveillance

Encryption, deep data, privacy, or cookie-consent forms bombard us online. Far from being free of surveillance today, we are induced to surrender to it fully.

One cause of our surrender lies in the enormous extent to which these technologies have made themselves an intimate and indispensable part of daily life. There is scarcely any place we can hide from this surveillance and still lead a normal existence (though a monastery on some Nepalese mountain top might just qualify).

In his writings, French sociologist and philosopher Michel Foucault noted how institutions like prisons and psychiatric institutions use

24-hour surveillance to control their inmates. This loss of basic privacy in every aspect of life conditions inmates to succumb more readily to authority. A similar means of control can be found in army boot camps, where not only is privacy surrendered but recruits must also wear the same uniforms, have their hair cut to the same length, accept daily parades and inspections—in short, endure a series of interventions intended to submerge their individuality and abandon any sense of control.

But these impositions are by design. Much of the surveillance we face today emerged innocently at first, and from there by almost unseen steps went much further. We are not, in the main, surveilled because we or anyone else wishes it (airport scanners and closed-circuit TVs are an exception). We are surveilled because we need the devices that contribute to this form of oversight and monitoring.

Today, we impatiently sign or click away whatever seems asked of us, following whatever search we find ourselves on. To this extent we seem to be living life through the screens of monitors, cell phones, iPads, and GPS guidance screens in our cars. The increasing ubiquity of mobile phones and tablets has made our screens much more than the portals they were once counted as being ("doors" as early writers spoke of these) and even more than "windows" as these meld with touch pads. There is also a tactile interface: swipe left, right, up, down, tap to localize, so the new advertising tells us, to infinity.

Screen-being is an imaginary projection, part of our endowment as conscious perceptual beings. But it is a learned projection, honed by film and television, by Google maps that can widen our sense of spatial being, and via GPS in cars. Whereas once our sense of self derived mainly from an inner world of thought and sensation, now we live with the direct consequences of having a cell phone in our hands almost constantly. Our need to sleep meshes conveniently with the need to charge the battery. Part of the ongoing millenarianism of our technocult era is that we now possess the virtual imagery required to suppose ourselves transhuman. The screen at our fingertips (and in our mind's eye) is the only ticket we seem to need for that imaginary achievement.

But with this mechanical expansion of our sense of self comes an invisible bubble of constant surveillance. We are photographed nearly all the time, mostly without our permission, mostly without our knowledge. And all around us are other humans preoccupied with their phones, unaware of or inattentive to us. This new technology not only makes surveillance an ever-present reality but also broadens the gaps between us. Just as we can reach out further into cyberspace, so we withdraw from contacts in physical space. There are serious consequences here for any society built on the premise of personal interaction.

We may be inured to this omnipresent surveillance, but that doesn't mean we can assume that our movements, interests, and activities are of little interest to certain others.[1] So far from disinterest, corporate entities seem keen to have us transfer whatever information they need to them, which we do every time we log into Facebook, Instagram, Twitter, WhatsApp, Snapchat, e-mail, what have you. And then there's GPS.

Most of us welcome this navigating technology. But it is more than that. If older generations listened to the radio in the car, and maybe even sang along, folks on road trips allow the GPS lady's voice (rarely a male voice) to be the soundtrack for hours on end. People even interrupt each other on such occasions, to be sure the GPS lady can chatter on undisturbed, even as she says the same thing again and again. We want to be sure we don't miss it, and in the process, we ignore one another. This is another destructive effect of what appears as an innocuous technology: it comes between us and even our closest companions.

Perhaps the intrusion of GPS navigation systems on road trip conversation seems a minor price to pay for safely arriving at one's destination.[2] Where things may be different are the ways GPS has changed dating and lifestyle, displacing certain set meeting spaces for romantic connection.[3] This has led to what some call a hookup culture, and certain researchers have pointed to a clear connection between dating apps and the closure of certain social meeting places[4] that formerly served gay culture along with the arrival of GPS with its indications of proximity. Of note, however, is that these same apps seem radically less helpful when it comes to discovering options for a long-term relationship.[5] Still, if what you want is a temporary hookup, these technologies work just fine, across the sexes and across orientations. At the same time, relevant to what we above called screen-being, some marketers have found an addictive feature to the action of swiping, and it has been argued that including features otherwise used in online gambling apps for cell phone dating apps is no accident.[6] The presentation of an infinite world of possibilities beyond the screen—just another click away, just another swipe away—is part of the addictive function of porn to begin with. The screen reinforces this.[7]

Fake News and the Post-Truth Blues

If the purpose of the Internet is to transmit information, the quality of this information is increasingly eroded to the extent that we are—not always in ways we notice—entangled in tinier and tinier bubbles of interest and personal focus. Whereas we once got most of our news from reliable outlets like the *New York Times* or the *Washington Post* or from TV networks such as CBS, today we get much of our news through the Internet. Depending on our browsing habits, this may include websites belonging to formerly all-print media, especially if you are either old or temperamentally politically conservative. But many Internet websites are the domain of narrowly focused writers with an ideology to disseminate, often with little or no editorial oversight to restrain dogmatic instincts. It seems plausible that the increasing gulf that separates right from left in our political arena may be due, in part, to the ability of Internet users to find confirmation of their particular beliefs and suspicions without being exposed to countervailing opinions.[8] Fake news, in this sense, is unbalanced news (if it is news at all). It is written to agitate, to foment controversy, to sublimate our natural desire as adult human beings to find consensus as a means of coexisting. Down this road lie some very dangerous trends. In the wake of what is called "post-truth," we have witnessed violent demonstrations, the public shunning of political figures and their staff, and even shootings.[9]

The Internet did not come into being to bring about this revolution in news reporting. But in the hands of ruthless propagandists or naive readers, it has become a threat to comity and self-control. The world can now appear as we wish it to be, facts notwithstanding. Of course, propaganda is scarcely a new phenomenon. In war, every combatant uses fake news to buoy up the troops and the folks back home. And dictatorial regimes invariably resort to this mechanism as a means of enhancing their power. The difference here is that the Internet has achieved a far greater reach than some tinpot dictator could imagine. And it has done so while indisputably enriching our lives, to such an extent that the cure (if there were one) might be worse than the disease.

Orienting Ourselves in the World

Apart from the threat of surveillance and fake news in the post-truth world, these new information technologies draw on the phenomenon psychologists call "accommodation." So ubiquitous are these new tools, we cease to pay attention to them to the extent that we no longer see them. That they do more than merely extend our senses has long been recognized. This extending of ourselves, backward and forward, projecting and retaining, is exactly what we as conscious, perceptual beings excel in. It is also how we manage to conduct job interviews via Skype and relationships via FaceTime, along the way bracketing the weird camera effects. But there are also more everyday consequences. Thus I relate a personal adventure with a certain device with a certain kind of touch screen, which I managed to lose late one New York evening. As soon as I realized I had lost it (almost immediately upon leaving the taxi), my concern—more like panic—was "security."

Like many users of technology, I regard security as a pain in the neck. I remain unpersuaded that one needs to change email passwords as regularly as university IT likes to force us to do, perhaps because I see limited appeal in reading someone else's email. But when my iPad went missing, I was of a very different mind. For an iPad is not a computer, as I try to tell people who are thinking of getting one. Nevertheless, iPads function in many ways "like" a computer. One can keep notes on it, which are also stored on the device, take photos, and so forth, which means that at any given time, an iPad can have a considerable amount of non-backed-up data on it.

I am an expert at losing my iPhone and my iPad in my own apartment. Thus I am also a practiced hand when it comes to the surveillance technology Apple builds into its machines, which can also be accessed on a PC. When my iPad appeared, dutifully blinking on a Google map somewhere in the Bronx, clearly still in the cab where I left it, I put it in lost mode and proceeded. My iPhone, which also tracked the device, insisted that the missing iPad was found. As the taxi made its way from fare to fare, I also received numerous falsely positive notifications to track and watch its travels.

There were two options: in addition to vicariously tracking my iPad, having put it in lost mode, I could enter my phone number and ask the finder to call me, all the while realizing that, this being a New York taxi cab, the odds of this happening were limited. Or, I could call the taxi driver's own surveillance agency, the taxi commission. Note here that I had no information other than the GPS data that was pinging my email regularly. I had no information about the cab except where it happened to be, because of the GPS data. Neither I did have the taxi medallion number, because I didn't take a receipt. And although I paid with a credit card, in the short term, this yielded no information.

What I did know was where the taxi had been and where it was currently, roughly speaking. As a native New Yorker, I was also aware that the driver records (and reports) pickup and drop-off locations and times. This I relayed to the commission and told them where the taxi was, reporting at intervals the taxi's current location. They coordinated the position of the taxi driver, and called him: Did he have a lost iPad in his cab? Yes, he said, it was right next to him, on the front seat. This led the dispatcher to suggest that the driver might drive, after asking me if I agreed to pay the fare, from his location to my house and return it to me. I happily agreed.

It was a little uncanny; like the voice of God, eyes from heaven seemed to be on the driver—as indeed, thanks to GPS, they were. And back he came with my iPad. I was very lucky, as I was planning on leaving town directly, so I thought to ask the driver to drive me to the airport a little earlier than I had planned, even though I had been up all night, simply to learn a little more about what had happened.

I discovered that the desirability of the iPad was also the very reason it could be found, as he had plugged it in, trying to get it to work, thereby keeping the battery on hours after the device should by rights have died. The driver hailed from the Ivory Coast, a nice guy; we talked (in French) about Brussels, where he had spent some time in the hotel industry and I some time writing my thesis decades ago, and I tipped him. A lot.

To summarize, mindful here that readers will have all the time in the world in which to draw their own conclusions, this chapter began with a reflection on the significance of screens and consciousness, reflecting on our absorption in the same, even to the most intimate degree. I noted the potential for near-universal surveillance that this new technology has brought with it. I observed the impact on dating culture for young people. And I pointed to the impact of these tools in the way we orient ourselves in the world.

But note the ambiguity in the term "tool." The dictionary defines "tool" as a device used to implement a task. In that sense, it is an instrument of the user. But what is unique about these new information "tools" is that we have, in an almost equal sense, become instruments of their use. We are thus better positioned to begin to understand what Henry David Thoreau said a century ago: human beings "have become the tools of their tools." That is both an intriguing and an ominous thought.

Notes

1. See, for one approach, using methodology taken over from another discipline, John Symons and Ramón Alvarado, "Can We Trust Big Data? Applying Philosophy of Science to Software," *Big Data & Society* (July–December 2016): 1–17; and see too Luciano Floridi, *The Ethics of Information* (Oxford: Oxford University Press, 2013), and Alexander Stingl, *The Digital Coloniality of Power: Epistemic Disobedience in the Social Sciences and the Legitimacy of the Digital Age* (Lanham, MD: Rowman & Littlefield, 2015).

2. However, GPS guidance reliability can be overestimated: see the introductory chapters to Greg Milner's *How GPS is Changing Technology, Culture, and Our Minds* (New York: W. W. Norton, 2017).

3. See, to begin with, Katina Michael and Roger Clarke, "Location and Tracking of Mobile Devices: Überveillance Stalks the Streets," *Computer Law & Security Review* 29, no. 3 (June 2013): 216–28; also see Jordan Frith, *Smartphones as Locative Media* (London: Polity, 2015) and Leighton Evans, *Locative Social Media: Place in the Digital Age* (Frankfurt am Main: Springer, 2015). Specifically, see Eskild Heinemeier, "Grindr has Changed Sex Culture among Gay Men: Dating Apps Have Changed the Rules of the Game," *Science Nordic*, October 13, 2017.

4. Hugo Greenhalgh, "Grindr and Tinder: The Disruptive Influence of Apps on Gay Bars: Dating Apps Mean LGBT People Do Not Need Physical Spaces to Meet One Another," *Financial Times*, December 11, 2017; cf., more recently still, "Meet Markets. How the Internet has Changed Dating: Better Algorithms, Business Models and Data Could Have Even More People Finding Partners," *Economist*, August 18, 2018.

5. Angela Watercutter, "Could a Text-Based Dating App Change Selfie-Swiping Culture?" *WIRED*, July 10, 2018.

6. See Nancy Jo Sales's HBO documentary, *Swiped: Hooking Up in the Digital Age* (2018). For a discussion, see Nathan McAlone, "The Journalist Who Provoked the Wrath of Tinder Is Back with an HBO Documentary That Shows the Bleak Reality of Dating Apps," *Business Insider*, September 10, 2018; as well as Carly Stern, "Eye-Opening Documentary Examines How Apps Like Tinder Have Fundamentally Changed Dating—And Provided a Forum for Abusive, 'Unacceptable' Behaviour," *Daily Mail*, September 11, 2018.

7. Thus Zoe Kleinman discusses the sensory effects of swiping in her BBC News Technology article "Are We Addicted to Technology?" *BBC News*, August 31, 2015. And see, related to the above reflections on the documentary *Swiped*, Eric Johnson, "Swiping on Tinder Is Addictive. That's Partly Because It Was Inspired by an Experiment that 'Turned Pigeons into Gamblers': Journalist Nancy Jo Sales Talks about the Gamification of Dating and Her New HBO Documentary 'Swiped' on the Latest *Recode Decode* Podcast," *Recode*, September 19, 2018.

8. See Nicholas Carr, *The Shallows: What the Internet Is Doing to Our Brains* (New York: W. W. Norton, 2010) in addition to Tim Wu, *The Attention Merchants: The Epic Scramble to Get Inside Our Heads* (New York: Vintage, 2017).

9. See here the contributions to C.P. Prado, ed., *America's Post-Truth Phenomenon: When Feelings and Opinions Trump Facts and Evidence* (Santa Barbara: Praeger, 2018) in addition to Steve Fuller's *Post-Truth: Knowledge as a Power Game* (London: Anthem Press, 2018).

CHAPTER SIX

Technology in the Hands of Children: Helpful Tools or Harmful Distractions?

Lisa Menard

We know that the brain is a delicate and complex organ. A child's brain in particular is even more fragile due to the rapid rate at which it is developing and interacting with the surrounding stimuli. From infancy, a young brain is absorbing everything, from basic colors and sounds to the more complex, such as language and appropriate behaviors and social cues. For thousands of years, all of the influences a child could be exposed to were arguably "natural." Colors and sounds came primarily from their immediate surrounding environment, whether nature or people. Emotional and social influences would come from immediate family and a surrounding community. It was an insular and limited experience by today's standards. Some would argue this was an archaic way of life and that we are all better off with our multitude of technological advances. After all, these advances have made life easier (in many respects), faster, and more efficient. Our world is certainly more connected on the surface. But for the developing mind of a child, is easier, faster, and more efficient an inherently good thing? Could it be that healthy development requires significant effort and time? If children are given electronic tools as soon as they are able to hold them or make them function effectively, they are arguably never being given the appropriate opportunity to learn that skill on their own, using their own minds to compute the answer, or their own hands rather than a computer. Socially, children now have access to the entire world; every culture and language is easily accessible online. Yet this connectivity is anything but intimate. It is carried out in private, through a screen, and bears no resemblance to an in-person, face-to-face interaction. In many ways we are just beginning to uncover the effects that rapid changes in technology are having on young users, and for all of the positives that technology brings, the effect on our children is cause for concern.

In 1980, in-home video game consoles became widely available in North America. Over the next decade, children, teenagers, and even adults no longer had to make a trip to the arcade, pockets full of quarters, to play their favorite games. By the 1990s, when the graphics of in-home consoles surpassed those of arcade machines, there was no turning back. What once was a social experience, a gathering place for like-minded video game enthusiasts and a social outing for a family or group of friends, had become a more individual experience, with participants becoming more socially isolated in order to enjoy this new prospect of partaking in video games at home.

By the 2000s, at-home video gaming saw yet another change in the introduction of the Internet. Graphics continued to improve drastically, and children could now interact with other players from around the world, adding a dimension of "reality" to the games. Playing against others without leaving the home also introduced a new realism in that these games could essentially be never-ending. Instead of single-handedly making their way through progressing levels in order to win, players now had dynamic interactions with other players, making each session uniquely different.

If none of this is alarming in the context of a single child who likely has other interests, consider that 98 percent of children under the age of eight have mobile devices at home—an increase from 52 percent only six years prior.[1] This alone might not be alarming, as the existence of a mobile device in the home does not necessarily mean those children have regular access to the device. However, the average time per day spent on those mobile devices has increased from 5 to 48 minutes, and 42 percent of these kids own their own mobile device, up from less than 1 percent in 2011.[2]

Is this even cause for concern? Is it plausible that a generation of young people who now have seemingly unlimited access to electronic devices is simply the way of the future, and not at all harmful? Perhaps this will simply create a wired generation who will grow up to work and live much of their day connected to devices. One could argue it's even a necessity. While a familiarity with the latest technology might very well be helpful and even a vital skill, there is compelling evidence that the significant increase in a more sedentary lifestyle that inevitably accompanies increased time on electronics is, in fact, detrimental to a child's physical and mental health.

Mental health issues have never been as prevalent as they are now. In fact, since 2006, emergency department visits for children and youth suffering from mental health issues have increased by a staggering 63 percent. Actual hospitalizations due to the same issues have increased 67 percent, whereas hospitalizations for all other conditions fell by 18 percent.[3] Discussions about mental health and the associated stigma are common, and society has come a long way in its understanding of mental health issues. However, an estimated 10–20 percent of Canadian youth are affected by mental illness, and Canada's youth suicide rate is third-highest in the industrialized world.[4] It is important not to quickly dismiss how an increase in youth screen time could be affecting young people. While it might be difficult to argue a direct correlation between the increase in use of electronic devices and an increase in mental health struggles in children, it is not as much of a stretch of the imagination to consider that an increase in an activity that typically does not include social interaction or, at times, any form of interaction could be harmful to one's mental health.

It is hard to ignore the impact that electronic devices are having on young people, considering it is now the norm for preteens and teens to have a variety of electronic devices and to be regularly engaged in their use. The use of social media apps alone has significant social implications for young people.

According to a 2017 report by the Royal Society for Public Health in the UK, social media platforms have been described as more addictive than cigarettes and have a varying level of detriment to a young person's mental health, including anxiety, depression, self-identity, and body issues.[5] According to the report, Instagram tops the list as the most detrimental social media app with regard to the impact on health and well-being. The Royal Society for Public Health is calling for changes to this type of social media app, including asking platforms to highlight when a photo, even one from a celebrity or fashion brand, has been digitally manipulated, arguing that young people, particularly young women, "are bombarded with images that attempt to pass off the edited as the norm.

This practice is contributing to a generation of young people with poor body image and body confidence."[6]

This lack of authenticity and false personas being put forward are further complicated by the intense social pressure created by these apps where posts and pictures need to receive sufficient "likes" by friends and acquaintances. New apps have been created to help users filter, buff, and edit out anything about themselves they don't want portrayed. It is the opposite of being confident in oneself and is the antithesis of a healthy self-image. It also creates an environment of judgment and of not measuring up that young people are not only figuratively, but also literally, carrying with them wherever they go.

The PEACH project, a study conducted in the UK, suggests that children who spend longer than two hours in front of screens have an increased likelihood of suffering from psychological difficulties such as behavioral, emotional, and social issues, regardless of how physically active they may be.[7] It suggests that while low amounts of screen time may not be problematic, the hours children are now spending in front of screens daily certainly seem to be. And while moderate physical activity did have a positive effect on psychological areas, overall, no amount of physical activity seemed to be able to compensate for high levels of screen time. "Watching TV or playing computer games for more than two hours a day is related to greater psychological difficulties irrespective of how active children are," said Dr. Angie Page, lead study author from the University of Bristol's Centre for exercise, nutrition, and health sciences.

Victoria L. Dunckley, M.D., argues that regardless of the presence of an underlying diagnosis such as depression or attention deficit disorder, successful treatment almost always requires elimination of electronic devices, often for several weeks. She refers to this as an "electronic fast" that is meant to allow the nervous system to reset itself.[8]

Her research has found that this not only increases physical activity in children but also can have other positive effects, such as improvement in mood, better focus, and deeper sleep.

Her argument sounds reasonable. Without the option of an electronic device for weeks at a time, children will have no other option but to engage in other activities that are bound to involve more physical and mental activity and, most likely, interacting with others. Realistically speaking, there are very few activities that a child could engage in as an alternative to an electronic device that wouldn't inevitably engage them in one of these healthier activities.

Take, for example, a puzzle. Though it might not require significant physical activity, it will require mental activity in a way that most electronic devices do not. But what about doing a puzzle on a device? Many parents feel that lengthy screen time is excusable, and possibly even positive and to be encouraged, if their children are engaging in screen time that is interactive, or educational in nature. However, Dr. Dunckley's research and experience seem to show the opposite. While there may be some obvious benefits to online learning, interactive screen time is more likely to cause sleep, mood, and cognitive issues due to the amount of hyper-arousal this type of screen activity causes. Quite simply put, children's brains are agitated due to the persistent high levels of arousal from too much screen time. Understanding this possibility does not require much of a mental stretch. Most adults could relate to this concept and have likely experienced a similar state of sensory agitation after many hours in front of a screen or other significant stimulus, such as a loud rock concert, sitting next to a screaming baby on a long flight, or another comparable situation in which the senses are overloaded for long periods of time.

Going one step further, not only is there evidence to support the detrimental effects of too much screen time on children's mental health, but there is an increasing trend of teenagers seeking professional treatment for what they would describe as a video game or Internet addiction.

While it is perhaps not yet classified as a recognized disorder, video game addiction is being treated as a legitimate addiction by many treatment facilities in North America, much like the treatment approach taken for addictions to pornography or online gambling. Last Door Recovery Centre in New Westminster, British Columbia, advertises that it offers a 90-day residential program for patients with drug, alcohol, video game and nicotine addiction.

This facility isn't unique. Similar treatment facilities across North America are treating young people for their video game and other online addictions due to a demand that seems to indicate that technology addiction can become as serious and detrimental as substance abuse. In the same way that a facility might treat substance abuse, technology addiction can be approached through similar steps, including assessments, a period of "detox," family support, and a treatment plan. Some offer nature-based retreats and opportunities to completely disconnect from our wired world and reconnect with nature. Perhaps the "archaic" ways of the past were better for our brains, even if they were not as convenient.

This nature-based approach is referred to as Wilderness Therapy. It is the intentional practice of removing sufferers from their addiction and placing them, quite literally, in the wilderness for extended periods of time. Run by traditional treatment facilities where the patient is in 24-hour care, the important difference is that for part of the treatment process, the "facility" is the outdoors, and therapeutic and educational programming is conducted in a wilderness setting.

Not only is this meant to remove the patients from access to or temptation from electronics, including everything from cell phones to computers, but it is intended to give the brain a chance to detox from the stimulus, or overstimulus, that a life centered around a dependence on electronics can create.

In 2016, Dr. Nicholas Kardaras wrote an article published in the *New York Post* titled "It's 'Digital Heroin': How Screens Turn Kids into Psychotic Junkies." The headline is shocking and perhaps even insensitive, but Dr. Kardaras is confident that his position is backed by science. "We now know that those iPads, smartphones and Xboxes are a form of digital drug. Recent brain imaging research is showing that they affect the brain's frontal cortex—which controls executive functioning, including *impulse control*—in exactly the same way that *cocaine* does."[9]

Although this is simply Dr. Kardaras's medical opinion, if he is correct in the existence of a correlation between increased screen time and executive functioning issues and challenges with impulse control, the natural question would be to ask is if too much screen time is in part to blame for the prevalence of attention deficit disorder.

To support this argument, a recent study published by the *Journal of the American Medical Association* suggests that adolescents who frequently use digital media may have increased chances of developing attention deficit symptoms.[10] The study looked at 15- and 16-year-olds with no attention deficit symptoms and followed any emergence of symptoms over a 24-month period. They found there was significant association between subsequent attention deficit symptoms and a higher frequency of digital media usage.

With advances in technology, today's electronic devices are also faster, more graphically superior and more stimulating to the senses than even a decade ago. With senses bombarded, it isn't difficult to imagine that young brains would be accustomed to these stimuli. If they are, then perhaps a brain that is not receiving the constant stimulus of an electronic device would find itself understimulated, bored, and lacking in attention.

While symptoms emulating a lack of attention span do not necessarily equate with an attention deficit diagnosis, the outcome is arguably still concerning. If young people have become accustomed to the stimulus and entertainment that electronic devices can bring, and in the absence of these devices, or perhaps even during their use, they seem to exhibit a lack of attention, poor impulse control, and poor executive functioning, it stands to reason that it is more important than ever to ensure that children are exposed to a multitude of stimuli, especially stimuli that do not come from the flickering of a screen.

If the brain becomes agitated and aroused in an unhealthy way, how then would this affect the ability to sleep? The importance of rest for all ages cannot be understated, but a child's need for sleep is different than that of an adult. Much of a child's cognitive and physical development takes place during those precious hours of deep sleep.

The blue light that is emitted from screens, while artificial, emulates daylight as far as the brain is concerned. When natural daylight fades, it is a trigger for the brain that it's time for sleep. With the creation of artificial blue light emitted from all the screens young people access, often until late at night and just before bedtime, the body's circadian rhythm is thrown off. According to the Harvard Medical School, light of any kind can suppress melatonin, a hormone that affects circadian rhythms, but blue light does so more powerfully. Compared to green light at a comparable brightness, blue light suppressed melatonin for approximately twice as long and shifted circadian rhythms by twice as much, according to a Harvard experiment.[11]

There are measures one can take to counteract the effect of blue lights, from avoiding screen time in the hours prior to sleep to the less straightforward option of purchasing blue light–blocking goggles. In addition, there are apps available that can be downloaded onto the device that will filter blue and green wavelengths at night. There is irony in the use of technology to solve the problems caused by technology.

If one were to momentarily suspend one's concerns over the myriad of potential effects or side effects of electronic devices on a child's mind, from a developmental or even mental health perspective, one must at the very least consider the physical effects of engaging regularly and repetitively in such a sedentary activity. The use of electronic devices is almost exclusively inactive from a purely physical standpoint. This translates to most children spending significant time simply not moving.

This new reality of inactivity is surely a contributing factor to rising obesity rates in children in Canada. The World Health Organization estimates that 31.5 percent of 5- to 17-year-olds are either overweight or obese.[12] Dr. Karl Kabasele, a CBC medical contributor, says that in addition to unhealthy eating, "kids are playing video games, watching TV, not getting out and exercising. So all of these factors are kind of conspiring against kids despite our best efforts."[13]

What's even more concerning is that the adult parents, who are arguably in control over the screen time of their children, are also battling with equally concerning obesity statistics. In 2015, 59 percent of Canadian adults were classified as either overweight or obese. This statistic does not include those adults who would be considered simply overweight but not yet obese.[14] This statistic is even more worrying when compared to 2003, when the obesity rate was only 14.5 percent.[15]

While obesity is not solely due to the prevalence of electronics in our lives, and the resulting increasingly sedentary lifestyle, the negative effects cannot be entirely discounted. Aside from obesity concerns and other weight issues, cardiovascular health can be affected when there is little activity. Children quite simply are not engaging in an active lifestyle at a young age and not learning the importance and good habit of making exercise a regular part of daily life. A simple and seemingly trivial example would be how children in the 1980s would hop on their bikes and ride through their neighborhood to their friends' houses. As they gathered at one house, their bikes would accumulate on the front lawn—a visual cue to other friends as to where everyone was gathered. It involved getting outside and riding or walking to meet up with their friends. Today's children would likely text each other or meet online. The dynamic has changed, and the ease that electronics bring to our lives naturally removes the effort. That effort was often physical, and while it may now be faster or easier, our ease comes at a price.

Even something as simple as the loss of the Saturday morning cartoons has an effect on the dynamic of choice for children. For decades, cartoons geared toward children were typically only shown on certain channels at certain times—like Saturday mornings. For many North American families, this would become part of their weekend routine. It was something children could set aside time for and look forward to—but more importantly, it was something they had to wait for. When the cartoons were over, and the programing switched to adult content, the children would need to move on to other activities. Further, the cartoons shown were at the discretion of the network or channel, and the children would have no control over programming. Simply put, they would get what they got. Their choice was to watch it, or choose a different activity—one that would arguably, at the time, not involve an electronic device. Fast forward two decades, and virtually any children's show is available at any time of day or night, on a multitude of devices (even at the same time), as long as the child's parents have purchased or subscribed to the required service. Is this convenient? Yes. Are options and accessibility progress? For the most part, yes. Does it benefit children to have access to whatever they want, whenever they want? Likely not.

The simple necessity of needing to wait (up to 7 days!) for a program they enjoy, teaches children patience—a trait that all children and adults will need daily for their entire lives. It teaches them that good things are worth waiting for, and most importantly, it allows them to enjoy something over which they do not have total control. This concept of "you get what you get" is not something that today's children often encounter as they exist in a world of access to whatever they want and need, often instantly.

The possible detrimental effects are significant and still very uncertain. With much of today's current technology being relatively new, and most certainly ever-evolving, it will be years, even decades, before long-term effects of the developing mind are fully explored. Despite these serious concerns, there are unmistakable benefits to technology that deserve both mention and consideration.

In an increasingly wired world and a world in which electronic options are sometimes the only option in particular situations, it is important to consider how beneficial technology can be in the hands of children and young people. There is no denying that technology has, in countless ways, made our lives easier, faster, more "connected," and more streamlined. Music and books, which normally would have been accessed in person, have even become "wired" and readily available.

Often, technology is being used by young people for educational reasons, rather than purely for entertainment or for social purposes. While many of the concerns previously mentioned, such as the dangers of the sedentary nature of sitting in front of a screen for hours per day would still apply, if the use of the screen was for educational purposes, are the benefits enough to balance out the potential dangers and detriments?

For adults, the benefits of technology are so common and prevalent that they are often taken for granted or are simply no longer noticed. In the context of children, looking at the ways they benefit from technology could help parents and educators find new ways in which to utilize technology and when to "turn it off."

If children are expected to be proficient in various forms of technology at school and most certainly in their future jobs, perhaps there is benefit to ensuring they have sufficient and regular access to a multitude of devices. Consider for a moment that if a young person had little to no awareness or ability to use technology, it would be considered outside of the norm. Society depends heavily on technology, from the simplest tasks to the most complex, and it seems that equipping our children with technological know-how is vital.

The simple ability to have instant access to information and knowledge is hugely beneficial. In a learning setting, both at school and at home, young people can have access to virtually anything in a few moments. Though certainly not as reliable or as trustworthy a source as perhaps an encyclopedia, the benefit is that electronic information has the capability of being updated, revised, and refreshed instantly—something an encyclopedia could not have been.

Most technology, and most certainly smartphones and computers, offers access to educational content. From practice tests and lessons to puzzles and problem-solving games, the opportunity for children to use technology for learning seems endless. Young people have an opportunity to teach themselves through the use of technology, rather than depending on a person or classroom setting to learn. While less social with regard to human interaction, the access to information provides a flexibility that offers almost total freedom to the user.

In this way, technology is beneficial to all children who can access it. Increasingly, its advantages can now extend to those who normally would not be able to access it, for example, a nonverbal child using technology to communicate for the first time. Not only does it provide a vehicle for communication but it can actually help children *learn* to communicate on their own. While a child without a disability might be able to learn a language through simply hearing it repeatedly over time, a child with a disability may only be able to learn words by seeing them and touching them. For some families, technology is the difference between a child who is thought to be unable to communicate at all and a child full of thoughts, feelings, and desires who merely needs a vehicle with which to express it all.

Dr. Stephen Hawking is one of the more eminent examples of how assistive technology can be used for communication purposes. Dr. Hawking communicated through the use of a variety of assistive devices after losing his ability to speak in 1985, following a tracheotomy and complications from his amyotrophic lateral sclerosis (ALS).[16] For close to 30 years, he used a computer-based communication system controlled by a hand-held clicker that allowed him to formulate sentences by clicking on word choices and commands on a computer screen attached to his wheelchair.[17] In 2008, when his muscle deterioration made his hand too weak to control the hand-held device, new technology allowed him to communicate through a device attached to the bottom of his glasses that would detect his intentional flexing of his cheek muscles. The sentences were then sent to a speech synthesizer. What would have been decades of being unable to communicate at all instead resulted in over 30 years of lectures, books, and other significant scientific contributions.

For children with physical disabilities, particularly those who do not have the use of their arms, technological advances in the area of eye-gaze technology now means that those same children can control a computer with only their eyes using eye movement and blinking. What once required a click of a mouse or a touch of the finger on a screen can now be commandeered by even very young children with an action as simple as holding their gaze on one spot on the screen for several seconds.

The benefits of technology for children who have a range of disabilities is indisputable. It's a testament to how far we've come with technological advances, and it would seem that we've only just begun to uncover how the lives of those with disabilities can be improved. But the reality is that the bulk of consumption of electronics by young people does not take the form of crucial assistive technology or educational programming. While these uses may be common and vital, the effects of technology and its excessive use by children for entrainment proposes serve little benefit but distraction. This is not to say that using technology for entertainment is inherently bad, but overuse is a concern, as is the lessening and loss of other interests or activities due to the increase in time spent in front of a screen.

The word "progress" is typically employed in a positive context. Culturally we view progress as constructive with an implication of moving forward toward improvement. When it comes to the speed and extent to which electronic devices have affected the daily lives of children, the "progress" made in this area is not necessarily having a positive effect when assessed overall. Neither is it exclusively moving children forward in a positive direction when the detriments are fully considered and weighed.

Although children most certainly need to be proficient in technology and be able to access a wide variety of devices for their future success, the copious amounts of time spent in front of screens at young ages, whether watching TV, playing video games, or partaking in social media, do not contribute enough toward any meaningful benefit that can be justified. This type of unnecessary or nonbeneficial usage by young people can be drastically reduced while still allowing them to access and enjoy using technology as a tool, rather than as their primary mode of entertainment. Children can still be tech savvy without being dependent on technology to fill their free time. The benefit of this approach means that the opportunity to explore, be entertained, and fill their time can be found outdoors with friends and family or even on their own, allowing the sights, sounds, and smells of their surrounding world to be their very best source of stimulation. At the very least, our children deserve an increase in the organic stimulations found only in the "real world" and a drastic decrease in artificial stimulation and simulation.

Notes

1. V. Rideout, *The Common Sense Census: Media Use by Kids Age Zero to Eight* (San Francisco: Common Sense Media, 2017).

2. Ibid.

3. Canadian Institute for Health Information, May 1, 2017, www.cmho.org /documents/CMHO_ED-Hospital Usage, 2017.

4. Mental Health Commission of Canada, *Making the Case for Investing in Mental Health in Canada*, 2013.

5. Royal Society for Public Health, #StatusOfMind—Social Media and Young People's Mental Health and Wellbeing.

6. Ibid.

7. Angie Page, "Screen Time Linked to Psychological Problems in Children," University of Bristol, October 11, 2010.

8. Dunckley, Victoria.

9. Nicholas Kardaras, "It's 'Digital Heroin': How Screens Turn Kids into Psychotic Junkies," *New York Post*, August 27, 2016.

10. Chaelin K. Ra, Junhan Cho, Matthew D. Stone, Julianne De La Cerda, Nicholas I. Goldenson, Elizabeth Moroney, Irene Tung, Steve S. Lee, and Adam M. Leventhal, "Association of Digital Media Use with Subsequent Symptoms of Attention-Deficit/Hyperactivity Disorder among Adolescents," *JAMA Network*, July 17, 2018.

11. Harvard Health Publishing, "Blue Light Has a Dark Side," https://www .health.harvard.edu/staying-healthy/blue-light-has-a-dark-side, August 13, 2018.

12. Karen C. Roberts, "Overweight and Obesity in Children and Adolescents: Results from the 2009 to 2011 Canadian Health Measures Survey," *Health Reports* 23, no. 3 (2012), 37–41.

13. Karl Kabasele, "31% of Canadian Kids Are Overweight or Obese," *CBC News*, September 20, 2012.

14. M. Tjepkema, "Measured Obesity: Adult obesity in Canada: Measured Height and Weight," *Statistics Canada*, Catalogue no. 82-620-MVE2005001.

15. "Statistics Canada: Overweight and Obese Adults (Self-Reported), 2014: Canadian Community Health Survey, 2003, 2005, 2007 to 2014," *Statistics Canada*.

16. Michael Courts and Sarah Keenihan, "A Timeline of Stephen Hawking's Remarkable Life," *The Conversation*, March 14, 2018 http://theconversation. com/a-timeline-of-stephen-hawkings-remarkable-life-93364.

17. Marco Grob, "How Intel Gave Stephen Hawking a Voice," *WIRED*, January 2015, https://www.wired.com/2015/01/intel-gave-stephen-hawking-voice/.

CHAPTER SEVEN

Learning in an Age of Digital Distraction: Education versus Consumption

Chris Beeman

Thought is changing. I do not mean by this that the subject of thought is changing, although this is probably also true, but rather that the process of thinking itself in this era we call digital is undergoing change. Along with this, the capacities for reasoned argument and reflection are also changing.[1] There is a corresponding pressure to transform educative practices. Many new strategies are geared to finding some way of holding the attention of an easily distracted group of students long enough for more complex thought to occur. (Try entering "maintaining student attention in a digital age" in a web search, and you might find an example as disappointing and digitally distracting as the one I encountered, which advocates giving up "complaining" about digital media and attempting to compete for attention through an amped-up kind of storytelling.)[2] The occasional calls for "critical thinking" notwithstanding, the whole project of public education is undergoing immense pressure to become yet another venue for the accumulation of more information, of data for public consumption.

This chapter makes the case that addiction to digitally gathered information, especially that found through social media, is changing what learning is understood to be, and with this change comes a need for educational responses that go beyond simply becoming more attractive in the same sense that digital information is. This chapter cautions against trying to compete by fighting fire with fire, as it were, when facing a Fire-Maker. It instead suggests a more careful consideration of learning in a broad sense and argues in favor of designing education more in keeping with a sense of inquiry. Ultimately, this leads to something like what has been described as *slow thought*,[3] but I am going to call it *intentional learning.*

If learning has itself changed, how has it changed? A relational and integrative approach was understood and honored in many Indigenous traditions[4] as well as ancient Western and Eastern ones. In such an approach to learning, at least a dialectical dance is permitted to unfold between what is known and already integrated and what is new and becoming integrated. The dance is never-ending because there is an infinite capacity to either understand and integrate or temporarily reject what cannot be immediately integrated.

A default setting for what learning consists in today much more closely resembles an absorptive, addictive consumption of digital information. That is to say, at least some aspects of learning have become like the one cigarette too many smoked by a true addict: consumed with disgust for the product, the process becomes self-disgust for having the addiction. And the cigarette—or digital bit of information—is finished with distaste, to be forgotten as soon as possible, until the next craving hits. As a digital parallel to the image now required by law to appear on cigarette packages, I imagine the bleary-eyed and sleep-deprived users who are unable to stop watching the next piece of breaking news or who have to wait up until they get a hundred likes on their posted photographs. Information whose automated delivery is regulated by algorithms that bear no ethical responsibility is delivered divorced from the relational context that gives tone, nuance, and, ultimately, meaning to it. And if it is accepted that the term accurately describes it,[5] this widespread addiction to digitally gathered information is changing what learning is understood to be in educative practice as well. Thus, the bulk of what learning has become has changed from a relational integration, as could be found in traditional Indigenous learning, to an all-absorbing, unquestioning consumption, as Carlos Prado suggests in his introduction to this collection.

A Bleak View of the New Normal Learning

Because of the availability of technology that makes acquisition of digital information easy and uncritical adoption of the norm, digital natives, such as those who now widely populate universities, are naturally inclined to think of learning as a reflex response to an external prompt, like snacking thoughtlessly while the movie plays on Netflix, or like seeing something appear in their inbox or newsfeed. The ding happens, and one looks at an inbox. This kind of learning has become automatic in the true sense: no intention to learn, no question to answer initiates it, and no action except a simple swipe is needed for this simple kind of consuming to occur. What makes it more complex is both the addiction to information acquired in this way and the algorithmic conjuring contained in apps that both make and intend to make these technologies and their concomitant information ever more addictive.[6] Because of the nature of the addiction to incoming information—an addiction promoted by those wanting to sell apps and devices (along with the attention of the very consumer using them)—and especially because their Facebook, Twitter, or other "feed" is designed to give them the kind of information they uncritically like, digital natives are likely to see any information that questions this model of learning, such as the kind of writing you are reading now, as foreign, intrusive, or perhaps as just feeling wrong.

A fair question is whether those with this addiction are capable of reasonably considering arguments against it. Certainly, most addicts are not moved by reasoned argument. Imagine trying to convince even a sober alcoholic, removed temporarily from his or her addiction—much less an inebriated one—why alcohol can be harmful. Why should the rewiring of the brain be any different? Or rather, why should the rewired brain have any capacity at all to understand the way of thinking employed by the brain that has not gone through such a radical connection between addiction and thought? Why should there be anything other than a sense that nothing is wrong, that this is the way the world is, especially when almost all other relatively privileged people in the world share the same addiction? If one is addicted to nonprescription drugs and almost no one else is, it is at least possible to look around to see others who appear to be happier and are not addicted. But if one is addicted to the same technology that almost everyone else is, then there is almost nowhere to look to find an alternative. Or perhaps the addiction is not to the technology per se, but, as with Gautama Buddha's insight, to the sensations produced in the body, and registered at an unconscious level,[7] through anticipation of, interaction with, and reflection on the events produced and largely controlled by the technology. Thus, it is not only that thinking is changing but that being is also.

The ease with which new information is acquired reduces the role of memory. What is carried with us, the pillars or supports upon which ideas are generated from within—or perhaps these are conduits through which they flow?—and upon which ethical decisions are taken, is almost nil. Our resources for critically placing, contextualizing, and judging new ideas are reduced. Even the need for short-term memory appears to be put into question by the way digital natives use technology. I have not done research in this area, but I have been surprised to see some signs of this. For example, some digital natives of my acquaintance appear to have a very strong attachment to precise web addresses when assigned web-based readings for courses. When readings are assigned, they may be seen making sure they get precisely the right address. This is stored. Once in possession, this code or key is often treated as being equivalent to the knowledge contained in the readings themselves. Thus, when a question is asked, digital natives can be seen scurrying to find an answer by finding the "code" to it: the digital address wherein the information is actually contained. The readings themselves have never been done. They don't need to be: what is needed is only knowing where to find the information when it is needed. There appears to be no cultural or ontological consideration given to the idea that we might become different kinds of people if we learn certain thoughts and carry them with us in the form of a changed being. Being able to find and access information has replaced actually reading, considering, and assimilating information and allowing it to be present and expressed as part of one's being. Of course, this is natural when there is simply too much information being thrown at one to have any hope of reading it, not to mention understanding it. In response to this need for more storage space, a cell phone has become an external brain, with immense storage capacity. And when a cell phone becomes an external brain, without a cultural understanding that this has happened, or that we want it to happen, or what as a culture we might do if this happens, an unauthorized and unconsidered position is automatically adopted. We simply do not know what will come about, not least to systems of democratic governance, when a person walks through the world without the kinds of background knowledge and shared ethical perspectives upon which to base everyday decisions.

In some Turtle Island[8] Indigenous cultures, creation stories offer everyday and more serious advice, with beloved animal spirits often taking the place of actors in dramas, whose characters put them face-to-face with dilemmas. Across several First Nations, Raven and Coyote are often in trouble. Their trouble results from often a human-like kind of cleverness that makes them wonder, question, and challenge. Great Spirit's helpers, whose names vary with the tradition (such as Napi Old Man in Blackfoot culture),[9] account for some of the mistakes made in creation.

In Keith Basso's wonderful *Wisdom Sits in Places*,[10] stories that are connected to distinct topographies in Western Apache lands inform ethical behavior and serve to aid in the education of younger members. In the story Basso tells, the acts of one person are referred to obliquely, as elders in the person's presence tell the ethical stories held by features of the landscape around them. There is never any direct disapproval expressed toward this person's actions; to do so would be to diminish him. But the characters contained in the land features are referred to, and he can make the connections himself with knowledge of his own behavior and actions. These stories are carried with the members of the nation. They are reinforced as the land is traversed. Each traveling through the territory has the capacity to cause a conscious or unconscious retelling of the stories. And the telling of the stories, as in Aboriginal culture in Australia, contributes to the singing into being of the world that the members of the longest continuous cultural tradition surviving today travel through: the Songlines. There is something about this integrated knowledge that some still move through the world with—a knowledge that one carries with oneself, constitutes oneself, or, more properly, a knowledge that creates the kind of being that is altered from one simply glimpsing the world that one passes through to one that creates a world of which one is a part.

There is also a crucial distinction between the kind of integrated learning that I mention just above and the kind of learning that occurs through an external prompt or from a device. I want to contrast a kind of mental process that is generated from within, in following a thought from beginning to end, in making an argument, or in telling a story that reaches the kind of ending, amorphous or clear, that is desired, with the kind of thinking that is merely or predominantly responsive to an external prompt (like a ding) provided by a nonhuman system. External supports such as land features—places one might travel to intentionally to be reminded of teachings—are quite different than repeated and almost limitless interruptions to thought that demand one's attention be drawn away from a task at hand and be devoted to a device with an apparent agenda of its own. In fact, the device does have an agenda of its own, which curiously, and not coincidentally, resembles what users themselves might have done to distract themselves. And this is because the actions the algorithms take are based on the predilections and psychological weaknesses of the user. I will note these in more detail in a later section. In summary, though, in spending time in the company of digital natives, I experience an immense capacity to become informed, in the sense of being able to sustain volumes of information being thrown at one, but relatively little skill in being able to formulate ideas generated from within.

What is worse, so many digital users glibly move from one frail idea to another, as their feeds tell them to. There appears to be no shame in telling the latest story, one that even a superficial analysis would show contradicts yesterday's—or yester-minute's—news that entertains, rather than bolsters, warns, informs (or *improves*, to use Jeeves's fortunate phrasing[11]). "News" takes the form of fashion and is mingled with gossip. It is entertainment, and this is partly why Trump, who a few years ago might have just been any fool, could get elected president. Once elected, the possibility for entertainment takes a quantum leap, and popularity consequently increases. The public sentiment that there is no more to any job than just playing a role is thus bolstered. And the show goes on. News, watched and cheered on in this way, becomes a political act as it is consumed; it contributes to reshaping the news cycle in ever more distressingly deviant ways, as reportage on significant and world-shaping events becomes entertainment in the most burlesque sense.

The kind of thought that analyzes, compares, finds patterns, imagines new ideas, discovers good arguments, finds out things—not that shock us from one moment to the next, but that rather lead us to unexpected and delightful new insights because it is predominantly self-generative— is lost in the fashion of the now and the instantaneous jolting of the moment. This ensures the continuation of consciousness from one moment to the next,[12] but the consciousness that continues is a misshapen and perhaps abused one, one that reacts and cringes, rather than one that is shaped gently by the having of wonderful ideas, to use Eleanor Duckworth's happy phrase.[13] For Duckworth, questions around "what if," or "I wonder if," are of the very stuff that constitute learning. In contrast to this, thought that is directed and controlled by the addictive algorithms of an external device is inherently reactive. The mind/body that is subjected to such continual shocking by external stimuli is one that is traumatized, rather than gently guided, into learning. The qualities of deep reflection, of fearless endeavoring to truthfully tell a tale, or to make an argument and refute it when that argument is mistaken, take a great deal of work and time to develop. Were it not so tragic, there is irony that at the time these qualities are most needed, there are fewer people developing them and far too few who understand the difference between them and the simple acquisition of random facts.

Why are cell phones so addictive? They are meant to be. From their use primarily as mobile telephones only a decade ago, cell phones have become the primary instrument through which digital information is consumed. Ira Basin's thoughtful Canadian Broadcasting Corporation (CBC) *Sunday Edition* radio documentary "Open to Persuasion"[14] makes a compelling case for why digital technologies are so demanding of attention. Once the user's attention has been captured, an addictive cycle ensues that makes getting out next to impossible. Basin also points to why these technologies are also so devastating in dismantling the undergirding necessary for democracy to survive: the ways information is provided through them takes away shared knowledge and replaces it with compartmentalized understandings of the world, which are subject to the personal preferences of the user. This section will refer in detail to Ira Basin's documentary in telling the story of why mobile devices are so addictive and persuasive in getting us to consume information and some of the effects of this addiction on democracy.

The reason mobile devices ("cells"), in particular, command attention is that both the cells themselves and the apps that you use on them are designed to do so. Communication with them is a by-product, with the real product being your attention, which is then sold to others in the form of providing a venue for advertising or information about the user. The science of commanding attention and of using this process to shape a user's behavior is called persuasive technology.

It used to be that television was an object of concern for its possible use of persuasive aspects to control us without our knowing it.[15] But then, the television was in the living room. It was turned on once a week to view special programs that families watched and perhaps even discussed together. Now we are being persuaded by cell phones, which are with us—literally on our person, to the extent that they become part of our person—all the time. In conjunction with the sheer amount of time we are in the grips of a persuasive technology, James Williams (with the Oxford Internet Institute), quoted in the documentary, notes also that what controls us is determined by fewer and fewer people. A handful of people can type a few keys and change a few algorithms, which in turn will choose which news articles go to which users, and change billions of minds. As Williams says, this is "a kind of persuasive power that is fundamentally new in history. . . . We don't even have a word for this type of persuasive power."[16]

Persuasive technology has been used for a very long time, though never as successfully as now. Starting with Packard's early work in the 1950s, noted above, it has come to refer mainly to the way digital technologies subtly manipulate, without users knowing how they are being manipulated. In 1998, B. J. Fogg came to head the Center for Persuasive Technology at Stanford University. His early insight was that in a digital world, persuasive technology would be everywhere. The story goes that he was excited about its power to positively influence people in areas like health.

As this chapter goes to press, for example, Manulife, an insurance firm, is offering reduced rates on insurance if the insured person wears a Fitbit with an app to track lifestyle choices.[17] And in this example lie both what have been considered the positive and negative aspects of persuasive technology.

Leaving aside for the time being the obvious critiques of even the "positive" aspects—that, in an extremely limited way, behaviors might be modified for better health, which include that behavior modification is being used at all, that privacy is foreclosed, that health might not be accurately described in the same way longevity is, that healthy choices might vary between people, and so on—the negative aspects are far worse.

B. J. Fogg warned against possible corporatization and that the evolution of persuasive technology ought not to be controlled by market forces. Fogg's insights included the idea that persuasive technologies would come to us in the ordinary course of our lives. We would not be aware that we were being persuaded at all. Obvious recent examples of this emerged in 2017, the attempts to influence both the Brexit decision and Trump's election. Millions of users simply thought they were getting news on their regular feeds, although in reality, their voting choices were being effectively manipulated, using psychological operations, or *psyops*, through the cooperation between Cambridge Analytica and AggregateIQ, with information provided courtesy of Facebook and other sources who had successfully gathered information about possible swing voters that was then used to *persuade* them.[18]

Now, people involved with persuasive technologies are speaking out. As James Steyer, CEO of Common Sense Media, notes, Fogg was effectively teaching techniques for keeping people addicted to technologies. "It's a business proposition. And they were taking advantage of the best, newest thoughts in psychology married to these new technology platforms that were completely unregulated."[19] Tristan Harris, who at one time held the somewhat fanciful title of Design Ethicist at Google and left it to form the Center for Humane Technology, noted that the psychological vulnerabilities of each user were being targeted with various enticing elements to addict him or her. Now Harris heads an independent think-tank that works in the opposite direction. He is convinced that persuasive technologies constitute an existential threat to the capacities and survival of humans. His argument is roughly as follows: Automated systems rank thoughts to put in front of a user. These systems are designed to capture the user's attention. What a given user sees, because of his or her psychological profile, is different from what others see. So, as nations and communities, we are fragmented into "echo chambers": we only hear what has already been said to *us*, and what others know we want to hear. Others hear versions of what has already been repeated to *them*. Thus, what would be usually called "Truth"—a relatively balanced version or events, or what most people would agree on if given similar information[20]—is utterly eradicated. There is no basis for enough commonality of understanding for discussions across the floor, as it were, with others holding deeply divergent views, when access to shared information—the ultimate irony in a digital age—is actually limited. If members of a given community or nation do not have shared information, leading to a possible agreement on truth, its members cannot agree on factual decisions to take on issues that affect the continuation of humanity. To wit: climate change and other current global threats.

Another knowledgeable critic is Sean Parker, the first president of Facebook. In describing early intentions in designing Facebook at a technology conference in Philadelphia in 2017, he said, "That thought process was all about how do we consume as much of your time and conscious attention as possible . . . that means we need to give you a little dopamine hit every once in a while because someone liked or commented. . . . The creators understood this consciously . . . and we did it anyway."[21]

While awareness of persuasive technologies increases, its use becomes ever more subtle and sophisticated. Nir Eyal, who studied with B. J. Fogg, works with developers with an interest in creating what he calls habit-forming products of the just the kind that Fogg expressed concern about and warned against. His vocation is reflected in the title of his book, *Hooked: How to Build Habit-Forming Products.*[22] In it, and in the seminars he runs for those designing apps, he outlines a four-step process through which attention is controlled. It begins with an external trigger like a ding sound. The prompt then tells you what to do next and requires an action, defined as the simplest thing done in anticipation of a reward. So, the ding teaches us to swipe our screen to see what has happened. Then a variable reward is given—the most effective way to continue to keep a person playing the game. The reward is based on the actions of users, from what they choose to do, to what they like, to what they post. These contribute to making the app better and better in the sense of occupying more and more of the attention (and time) of those consuming it. This is the investment phase of the cycle. An app's ability to addict is further strengthened by incorporating information derived from how each user interacts with the system. And the information users provide, such as posting on Facebook, not only gives feedback to the controlling corporation but also makes the addiction more potent to other users. This model of addiction leading to more addiction is an almost perfect business model.

There is a still darker dark side: to be really hooked, the user needs to be motivated by internal, not external, triggers. Specifically, negative emotions are very influential. So, an app that is successful at being addictive preys upon (my language) normal, usual, everyday negative emotions such as loneliness, sadness, or boredom. When the user is lonely or bored, the user learns to check Facebook. The pattern of a given user can become better and better known in advance by taking account of users' prior actions. And the "service" they use sells their information to others while their attention is held, and it is capable of learning their patterns and shaping what it gives them at different times each day, each week, each month, as their patterns become known and capable of being manipulated by powerful algorithms.[23]

Education as Consumption

Given the amount of time users spend each day being linked to a device and being schooled through addictive technologies, learning itself has changed. Thus, what is seen as "learning" today appears to be broadly linked to consumption of information, which is, in a sense, force-fed through the power—psychologically validated—of social media and the addictive quality of the devices themselves. As with anything consumed, at some point it is incumbent on the consumer to ask if his or her patterns of ingestion are healthy or destructive. I argue the latter. And I argue that educational responses have lost their footing in knowing how to respond: education has become a form not of learning how to think in certain ways that are germane to the discipline but of ingesting, at ever more rapid rates, information, sometimes with educators feeling the need to compete (of course, failingly) in the ways digital information is consumed.

I want to move from this idea to exploring the meaning of consumption itself. I am concerned that learning and, de facto, education, if left uncritically examined, will come to behave in similar ways to the way the terrible illness of tuberculosis was described in early times.[24] Even in the earliest descriptions, it was noted that patients were more and more consumed by the illness. They appeared to be being reduced, and *indeed consumed*, by it. Addictive technologies have come to dominate our minds through the forced need to ingest more and more information. Thus our limited mental resources come to be consumed, just as tuberculosis was thought to come to dominate the body through the *consuming* of all of its resources. In both cases, the person is consumed by the illness. As we become more information-saturated, we become less informed. As we become less informed, we become less knowledgeable and less skillful.

And as we become less knowledgeable and less skillful, we lose the muscle memory of critical awareness and consideration that characterizes intentional learning. Our ability to discern diminishes; thus our systems of government falter, and our ability to act collectively and effectively disappears.

As the addictive substance is consumed, so it consumes its consumer. It might be argued that there is a need for a frank encountering of digital information and the technologies that provide it with an understanding of it as being the most addictive of substances, precisely because its lack of physical form makes it all the more potent. When it is information and the delivery devices themselves that are the addiction, the instantaneous nature of the hit means that it is even more powerful than drugs that require the addition of a physical substance to the body. And the aspect of the person that is consumed through digital technologies is that which has to do with thinking, as it comes from within the thinker. The kind of thinking, which is only responsive to an external stimulus and quickly dies without it, is not the kind of thinking that will enable people to continue to adapt and thrive.

Knowledge Isn't Like That

Knowledge can never be simply accumulated without some kind of organizing system. Dewey recognized this and argued for a certain kind of organizing, one that recognized the similar interests between problem solving, what he called *growth*, and democracy.[25] Paulo Freire, in working in adult literacy with campesinos in Brazil, realized that there was no such thing as a neutral text: information always requires some organization, and the kind of organizing system may shape not just language ability but also progressive aspects of a citizen's character. So, Freire's teaching of literacy with the groups he worked with came to be based on socialist principles that could shape their lives for the better. Yet the predominant organizing system for knowledge is now an algorithm, without the intent of promoting learning but rather of increasing profit through controlling consumers' attention and selling this attention and its concomitant personal information to advertisers and other corporations. Citizen has become guinea pig; learner has become consumer.

In theory, the most basic system of organizing information would be simply additive. Some would argue that this kind of system would be neutral. This is a kind of organization that would not be possible in a nondigital age. But it becomes possible now: think of how convenient it is to deliberately not make folders to organize one's email account because to do so would require one to remember which folder the email was put into. Rather, it is much easier now to simply search the entirety of an inbox when an email needs finding. And every more powerful computing system makes possible the retrieval of information with only the most tenuous recollection. In an additive system such as an inbox, one piece of information is simply added to another piece.

But sometimes information is, significantly, not able to simply be added: for this to occur, other information would have to be found to be untrue. For example, if I add the fact that certain cancers are influenced by bacteria to already existing knowledge about these cancers, then an underlying thesis that cancer growth is genetically determined is at least challenged and perhaps diminished. I cannot maintain all competing theories for it, because the presence of one implies the reduced effect of the other. Algorithms designed to hook your immediate attention are not good at deciphering meaning and recognizing compatibility; they are good at simply adding stuff. Thus, if the algorithm for digital arrangement of information is simply additive, with no allowance for the almost infinite capacity of computers to store information, which is something distinctly different from the way the human brain has been organized over eras of human history, then this can be the basis for shifting what knowledge means. Knowledge can come to mean simply more facts added to an already overflowing base of facts. Somehow the truth is expected to emerge from these, in the same way one can imagine the popularity of given posts being determined. Simple likes or their absence do not accurately do this, though, when more complex ideas are to hand. For a computer, "truth" might emerge from a stack of facts. For a human, it will not; note the common legal trick of swamping the opposing party with banker boxes of files just before a hearing and being able to claim that supporting documentation was provided. In such cases, while it is true that information had been delivered, it is equally true that the information is inaccessible, that its import is not able to be discerned, if only because not enough time has been allowed for its digestion—information that is not given time to be digested not only causes indigestion, it misleads. It appears to mean something that it does not, and it leads in directions that are not legitimate. Thus, there may be a theoretical discrepancy between the kind of information that can be used by computer programs and the kind that is useful to humans. Yet we are living in a world in which the two competing interests are considered compatible. Not only this, but of course, information is not just added. Algorithms designed by people intending to make a profit choose which information a user has access to and which not.

Intentional Learning

In the new context of learning whose default setting is more like what computers do, learning needs to become, again, an intentional act. Perhaps to even have to make this statement is an ironic act, because what is being suggested is that we just learn the way humans always have. Yet in this particular era, in at most a couple of decades, the transformative effect in both behaviors around learning and in states of being influenced by these has changed so radically that we really do need to think about learning as an intentional act.

I would like to contrast my notes above on the change in what now tends to constitute knowing, learning, and information acquisition with what might be called intentional learning: engaging in the complex learning dance between what is known, considered, and part of a repertoire—a bundle, to use the English translation of the Anishinaabemowin term—and what is encountered. In this sense, the term "slow learning" is accurate. A conscious deliberation of new ideas and bringing them to the body of the old, which is contained in the body of the person learning, is an aspect of this. This is done knowing that what unfolds cannot be anticipated and will not always be pleasant—though the overall trajectory will most definitely be so. Even this dance is now in grave danger of being taken over by an overbearing partner who thinks it knows which way both dancers should move: the partner of instrumentalized learning, so common today in educational theory, in which every educative move is expected to produce a particular outcome. I recently heard tell of a teacher in early grades in the public system in Ontario whose practice was criticized by specialists who entered her classroom. They chastised her for not knowing the precise learning outcome that could be attached to the pile of rocks she kept handy for free and creative play. In the view of the specialists, every single event was to have a predictable and knowable outcome. That is not the kind of dance to which I am referring—a regimented march of predictable steps.

The dance I am referring to can either have an external instructor or come from within the learner. It is an unfolding of the unexpected with only a broad and overall intention to start off in a certain general direction, as any dance is. Something like the sentiment, "I think this looks interesting . . . let me go here," is its beginning point. It is learning based on hunches, with these becoming ever more accurate as the dance is danced. The learning dance I am referring to does not know what will happen in advance, does not know its "learning outcomes." It is a new dance in the mind of each student, and it happens impromptu always, as a person meets a subject and gives oneself over to the subject while simultaneously reveling in its plenty. However, the limitations of space determine that a fuller exploration of this be part of a later work.

Notes

1. Please see, in an earlier volume, Chris Beeman, "Do Social Media Interfere with the Capacity to Make Reasoned Arguments?" in C.G. Prado, ed., *Social Media and Your Brain* (Santa Barbara, CA: Praeger, 2017).

2. "The Alchemy of Attention: Four Strategies Storytelling in the Digital Age," 2018, https://medium.com/digital-learning/attention-and-the-alchemy-of-storytelling-in-the-digital-age-fe2b6204bebd.

3. Vincenzo di Nicola, "Slow Thought: A Manifesto," 2018, https://aeon.co/essays/take-your-time-the-seven-pillars-of-a-slow-thought-manifesto.

4. J.R. Miller, *Shingwauk's Vision: A History of Native Residential Schools* (Toronto: University of Toronto Press, 1996), pp. 18–38. In *Shingwauk's Vision,* John Miller gives examples of ways ethical behavior was, precontact, fostered in young Indigenous people through ceremonies such as the *walking out* ceremony, in which children symbolically performed actions that represented acts of service to their communities.

5. Evidence for this claim is presented later in the chapter.

6. Ira Basin, "Open to Persuasion: You Can't Stop Checking Your Phone, because Silicon Valley Designed It That Way," *The Sunday Edition*, Canadian Broadcasting Corporation, September 8, 2018, https://www.cbc.ca/player/play/1320657987764.

7. A synopsis of Gautama Buddha's psychology is contained in William Hart's book, *The Art of Living: Vipassana Meditation* (New York: Harper Collins, 1987).

8. The name for what is now referred to geographically as North America, but more with the sense of a home with a history.

9. For children's level introductions, see Paul Goble's *The Earth Made New* (Bloomington, IN: World Wisdom, 2009).

10. Keith Basso, *Wisdom Sits in Places* (Albuquerque, NM: University of New Mexico Press, 1996).

11. Jeeves, faithful servant and far superior thinker than his bumbling employer Wooster, sometimes admits to reading *an improving book* once his duties are done and before retiring. P.G. Wodehouse, *The Inimitable Jeeves* (London: Herbert Jenkins, 1923).

12. Hart, op cit.

13. Eleanor Duckworth, *The Having of Wonderful Ideas* (New York: Teachers College Press, 2006).

14. Basin, op cit.

15. Vance Packard wrote about this in 1957 in *The Hidden Persuaders*. Packard's work is described in the documentary by Basin, noted above.

16. Op cit.

17. Pete Evans, "Manulife to Offer Canadians Discounts for Healthy Activities," *CBC News*, October 2018, https://www.cbc.ca/news/business/manulife -fitness-insurance-1.3439904.

18. Carole Cadwalladr, "The Great British Brexit Robbery: How Our Democracy Was Hijacked," *Guardian*, October 2018, https://www.theguardian.com /technology/2017/may/07/the-great-british-brexit-robbery-hijacked-democracy.

19. Basin, op cit.

20. Of course this claim is open to challenge. Employing the principle of charitable interpretation, I would understand this as a Pragmatist approximation of Truth, rather than an attempt to invoke Truth in an absolute sense.

21. Basin, op cit.

22. Nir Eyal, *Hooked: How to Build Habit-Forming Products* (Penguin: Portfolio), electronic edition, https://www.amazon.ca/Hooked-How-Build-Habit-Forming -Products-ebook/dp/B00HJ4A43S. Also, a YouTube video is available at: https:// www.youtube.com/watch?v=hVDN2mjJpb8.

23. Basin, op cit.

24. C. Koehler, "Consumption, the Great Killer," October 2018, https://pubs .acs.org/subscribe/archive/mdd/v05/i02/html/02timeline.html.

25. John Dewey, *Democracy and Education*, Project Gutenburg, 2008, Ebook #852, https://aeon.com/essays/take-your-time-the-seven-pillars-of-a-slow -thought-manifesto.

CHAPTER EIGHT

The Kids Are All Right: Lessons from the March for Our Lives

Jason Hannan

In 2017, LA Reel House Media released a satirical YouTube video titled "A Millennial Job Interview."[1] The video begins with a middle-aged man interviewing a young Millennial woman named Amy for some unspecified job. He asks Amy whether she is adept at Excel. Amy is obnoxiously busy texting, too preoccupied even to look up from her phone. She rudely and impatiently says, "No." The interviewer then asks her about PowerPoint. In the same rude, insolent tone, she says, "No." He asks her about Microsoft Publisher. Again, "No." Exasperated, he then asks Amy in what applications she *does* hold some proficiency. Like a clueless and utterly vacuous airhead, she proudly replies, "Snapchat, Pinterest, Instagram, Vine, Twitter. You know, the big ones!" When facetiously asked about Facebook, Amy laughs and says, "That's for old people. Like my parents!" The remainder of the video continues to depict Amy as arrogant, self-entitled, lazy, and grotesquely incompetent. She is so lazy and incompetent that she relies on Siri to do her thinking for her. She refuses to come in to work at 8:00 a.m., insisting she's a late sleeper who doesn't even order her absurdly complicated Starbucks latte until 10:00 a.m. When told she's not the right fit for the job, Amy gets triggered, displaying extreme emotional fragility. She demands to speak with an HR represen-tative. In the end, the only way to convey to Amy that she isn't getting the job is for her to be told that she's fired. Amy leaves in disbelief and disgust.

As of this writing, "A Millennial Job Interview" has been viewed 5.7 million times on YouTube and over 25 million times on Facebook. Its astonishing viral success is a testament to the popular narrative about the supposedly sad and sorry state of young people today.[2] This narrative comes in different variations but nonetheless takes a common form. Typi-cally, it characterizes young people today as a pathologically inept genera-tion, owing to helicopter parenting and smartphone addiction. We are to understand that today's youth, having been coddled from birth and raised in front of screens, have grown up to be incredibly naive, presumptuous, and self-confident. They feel entitled to life's many rewards and riches despite never having worked hard enough—or at all—to deserve any of it. They feel entitled to everything from good grades and teacher praise to a college degree and a good job after graduation. When they don't get what they want, they pout and whine and complain. Because of a child-hood of ceaseless pampering and coddling, they can't handle criticism or even challenging ideas. They get too easily triggered and threatened and therefore require trigger warnings and safe spaces for their protection. Worst of all, they are hopelessly dependent upon smartphones and social media. They have the attention span of a gnat, the maturity of a child, and the vanity of a runway model. Young people, we are to believe, are woe-fully incapable of making their way in the world save through the medium of an iPhone. They rely exclusively on digital technology to think, to com-municate, to act. This addiction to technology has left them effectively handicapped. They text; therefore they are. Deprive them of their iPhones, and they will cease to exist.

This insidious narrative seems to have exerted such a powerful grip upon the popular imagination that young people themselves can be for-given for believing it.[3] It's an appealing narrative to Baby Boomer parents, high school teachers, university professors, and political ideologues of various stripes. Indeed, blaming or pitying young people has become such an ingrained cultural habit that we now take it for granted that there's something wrong with them. But is there any logical basis for this habit? Is the popular narrative about young people *true*? Does this sad, pathetic portrait bear any resemblance to actual youth today? Are they really the delicate "snowflakes" they are so often made out to be? Are they really that arrogant, naive, and self-entitled? Are they really as shallow and one-dimensional as the fictional Amy in the satirical video? Most importantly, is their supposedly pathetic condition the result of a collective addiction to smartphones and social media?

The purpose of this chapter is to question this insidious, condescending narrative of today's youth as the coddled, entitled, lazy, fragile generation. I challenge this narrative through a case study: the #NeverAgain movement and the March for Our Lives, a historically unprecedented response to gun violence in America. Led by teenagers, the #NeverAgain movement and the March for Our Lives not only changed the national conversation about guns but also achieved the unthinkable: putting the National Rifle Association, once thought to be invincible, on the defensive. As I argue below, the #NeverAgain movement and the March for Our Lives demonstrate two things. First, today's youth do not fit the negative stereotype crystallized in the "A Millennial Job Interview" video. On the contrary, they have proven themselves to be politically savvy and culturally attuned. Second, digital technology, far from being a social, intellectual, and emotional crutch, has proven to be an effective tool for political organizing by those intelligent enough to wield its powers. Against the popular narrative about today's youth, this chapter adopts a more nuanced stance that views technology through the dual prism of power and resistance.

Teenagers, Technology, and Technological Determinism

Of the many alarmist reports over the last decade about the supposedly catastrophic effects of smartphones upon teenagers, one that stands out is Jean Twenge's "Have Smartphones Destroyed a Generation?" which appeared in the September 2017 issue of *The Atlantic*.[4] An adapted excerpt from her book, *iGen: Why Today's Super-Connected Kids Are Growing Up Less Rebellious, More Tolerant, Less Happy—and Completely Unprepared for Adulthood—and What That Means for the Rest of Us*, Twenge's article is an extreme example of sensationalist pop psychology that does more to obfuscate than to enlighten. Twenge contended that a significant shift occurred with the introduction of the smartphone into our culture. While the pre-smartphone generation did grow up in front of screens, mainly owing to computers and the Internet, Twenge contended that teenagers today have grown up specifically on smartphones and social media, thereby being socialized into the world in an altogether different way. Teenagers today, she observed, are more shy and antisocial. They are less likely to go out on dates or to indulge in sexual activity. They have no desire to drive a car. They drink less and party less. "So what are they doing with all that time?" Twenge asked. "They are on their phone, in their room, alone and often distressed."[5] Teenagers today are more vulnerable than teenagers of the past. They are more prone to depression and suicide. While their lack of interest in driving, partying, drinking, and sex is good news for their parents, Twenge warned that teenagers today have become so dependent upon smartphones that they are too handicapped to handle real-world, adult challenges like getting a job.

Twenge's widely circulated and much-discussed article is a stark example of technological determinism. At its core, technological determinism is the view that technology drives culture, society, thought, discourse, language, and values. It posits that technology holds a special power to cut through the conservative forces of tradition and to revolutionize the way people make sense of the world; the way they relate to each other; and the terms on which they think, speak, and act. According to this view, technology's march through history cannot be traced to any one conscious will or intention; rather, technology functions as an independent and supraconscious force, one far beyond the deliberate choices of any specific individual or group.

Theories of technological determinism can be found in different schools of thought. As a historical materialist, for whom history is powered by the material conditions of society, Marx regarded technologies of production as the material basis for the cultural and intellectual superstructure of society.[6] The Toronto School of Media Theory held that media forms were the primary influence upon cultures and civilizations. Harold Innis argued that the dominant medium of a society holds a "bias" that determines the nature of that society.[7] Similarly, Marshall McLuhan argued that the key to understanding a culture lies in its dominant media forms: that once we understand the nature of those media, we will be able to understand the nature of the culture to which they belong. Hence we have McLuhan's celebrated aphorism, "The medium is the message," according to which the study of media forms is more profitable than the study of media content.[8] In a similar vein, Neil Postman has argued that television has revolutionized society, such that public discourse now takes the form of entertainment.[9]

While there is considerable merit to the view that technology shapes culture, the danger lies in generalizing about the effects of technology and reaching absolute conclusions. It is a very short step from asserting that technology holds culture-transforming power to concluding that technology is all-powerful. The danger of making this leap is that it leaves no room for resistance and fails to account for empirical counterexamples that defy the supposed omnipotence of technology. This leads to the more nuanced view of technology by cultural theorists such as Andrew Feenberg and Douglas Kellner, who view technology as holding both repressive and emancipatory potential.[10] According to this line of thought, it is not a given that technology should have this or that effect upon society, especially a negative one. All effects are the result of political and economic forces that can be either managed or resisted. Feenberg and Kellner are thus proponents of democratizing technology so that it serves the benefit of the public rather than the interests of a relative handful of wealthy and powerful elites. From their critical standpoint, the danger of Twenge's argument is that it attributes far too much power to technology, that it regards smartphone technology in particular as having an inevitably negative effect upon teenagers, and it regards teenagers as essentially lacking in the powers of critical thinking and political resistance. Hence, we are left with an utterly bleak and depressing portrait of mutant humans, zombies sitting in the dark staring into a screen, fated to remain forever helpless. The problem with this view of technology and teenagers is that it cannot explain the historic events that followed the horrific mass shooting at Marjory Stoneman Douglas High School.

The New Columbine

On February 14, 2018, 19-year-old Nikolas Cruz entered the grounds of Marjory Stoneman Douglas High School in Parkland, Florida, armed with an AR-15–style rifle he had legally purchased from a local gun store. Cruz, who was known to his peers to be mentally disturbed and badly in need of anger management counseling, opened fire upon a group of Stoneman Douglas students, killing 17 of them and injuring 17 more.[11] After leaving the campus and going first to a nearby Subway and then to a McDonald's, Cruz was soon apprehended and eventually confessed to the shooting. On March 8, 2018, Cruz was indicted on 34 counts of murder.[12]

The Stoneman Douglas massacre became the deadliest school shooting in U.S. history, surpassing even the Columbine massacre, which had come to occupy a special place in the American social imaginary, due in no small part to Michael Moore's blockbuster documentary *Bowling for Columbine*. After a long string of deadly mass shootings across the country, the Stoneman Douglas massacre proved to be a tipping point not just for the country, but especially for the students who had survived the massacre and had just lost their friends. Fed up with the alarming and shocking rate of national gun violence; the lobbying, bullying, and intimidation tactics of the NRA; and the lack of political will or even desire on the part of their elected representatives to take action, the students of Marjory Stoneman Douglas High School took it upon themselves to fight back. Their activism may prove to be a historical turning point for the United States.

#NeverAgain

Following the tragic shooting at Stoneman Douglas, a group of courageous and determined students decided to take their future into their own hands. This group was led by Alfonso Calderon, Sarah Chadwick, Jaclyn Corin, Ryan Deitsch, Emma González, David Hogg, Cameron Kasky, Delaney Tarr, and Alex Wind. They started the hash tags #NeverAgain and #EnoughIsEnough, effectively launching a revolution on social media.[13] Their personal Twitter accounts attracted hundreds of thousands of followers. David Hogg soon amassed over 800,000 followers on Twitter, and Emma González, over 1.6 million. Both surpassed the following of the NRA—González doing so in less than two weeks.[14]

Three days after the shooting, González delivered a powerful, nationally televised speech, which sent shockwaves around the country.[15] Using clear words, graphic imagery, and emitting raw passion, González managed to capture the mood and spirit of millions of Americans. She criticized the media for hounding the students, hovering over the school by helicopter, exacerbating their trauma and anxiety. She criticized certain voices in the news media and on social media for suggesting that the students were to blame for not having reported Nikolas Cruz earlier for his mental health problems. She forcefully subverted this twisted logic by adamantly condemning the egregious moral fallacy of blaming the victims. Turning the tables, she took to task all those who knew about Cruz's love of guns—his friends, family, and neighbors—but who never did anything about it. She took to task a legal system that allows a mentally ill teenager to purchase a military-style semiautomatic weapon. She called out corrupt politicians who, in routine fashion, offer "thoughts and prayers" after each mass shooting, followed by absolutely no meaningful action. She called out the National Rifle Association, condemning it for donating millions of dollars in financial support to politicians. She even went so far as to calculate how much each dead student was worth by donation numbers. González went further and called out President Trump himself, harshly criticizing him for repealing an Obama-era rule that made it more difficult for people with certain mental health problems to obtain a gun. She displayed a remarkable understanding of the politics of gun control, especially of Republican opposition to legislative reform.

She criticized Iowa Senator Chuck Grassley for blocking a mechanism that would have reported those receiving disability benefits for mental illness to the FBI's background check database.

In one of the most memorable parts of her speech, González went after "companies trying to make caricatures of the teenagers these days, saying that we are all self-involved and trend-obsessed and they hush us into submission when our message doesn't reach the ears of the nation."[16] She went through a long list of false and obnoxious talking points, from politicians to the media to Second Amendment fundamentalists, calling "BS" on all of them. Most importantly, she called "BS" on the popular myth that "us kids don't know what we're talking about, that we're too young to understand how the government works. We call BS." Through her powerful oratory, González inspired millions of young people across the country to join the national movement for gun control. The visual image of a fiery young Latina with a shaved head served as a powerful counterpoint to the image of prim and proper white male politicians who mindlessly recycle talking points handed to them by the industries who have bought them out.

On February 18, 2018, Parkland student Delaney Tarr published an op-ed piece in *Teen Vogue* titled, "I Survived the Parkland Shooting. This Is What I Want Everyone to Know."[17] Amid the media publicity—the good, the bad, and the ugly—Tarr reminded everyone that the survivors of the Parkland shooting had just lost their childhood. "The regular, ordinary concerns of high school students," she said, "are now gone for myself and my fellow classmates." Tarr went through a list of ordinary concerns of typical teenagers, such as class projects, finding a prom date, and planning a trip after graduation, activities that are no longer a part of her everyday preoccupations. Instead, she pointed out, she is now preoccupied with the fight for gun control and with making sure that every child, "every person, deserves to feel safe wherever they go, especially at school." She acknowledged that her newfound platform signaled both the abandonment of her youth and also the incredibly important responsibility of speaking out against gun violence and fighting for change.[18]

On February 20, 2018, Parkland student Cameron Kasky wrote an op-ed piece for CNN entitled, "My Generation Won't Stand for This."[19] Kasky recounted what was supposed to have been a normal day at school but which turned into a nightmare. He guided the reader through the harrowing experience of living in the midst of a mass shooting, not knowing what was happening, and learning that many of his friends were killed. Translating his pain and suffering into a direct call for action, Kasky wrote, "We can't ignore the issues of gun control that this tragedy raises. And so, I'm asking—no, demanding—we take action now."[20]

Alfonso Calderon traveled with a group of Parkland student survivors to Tallahassee, where he urged Florida legislators to take action and enact gun reform immediately. In a publicly televised speech, Calderon spoke about hiding in a closet for hours with his friends while they cried on to his shoulders, fearing for their lives. He spoke about the emotional pain of having to say good-bye to his parents by text, as he thought he might not make it out alive. He rejected the belief that teenagers can't be taken seriously because they're teenagers, and that his pain and anguish, his anger and determination, can't be as genuine and as valid as those of an adult. Calderon spoke on behalf of children everywhere, insisting the time had come for everyone to listen to what the children had to say. He made it clear that they wished to live and that they would do everything they could to mobilize and to fight for their future.[21]

One of the most prominent voices to emerge from Marjory Stoneman Douglas was David Hogg. A mature, confident, articulate, and charismatic speaker, Hogg became a strong presence on the news media and on social media after the launch of the #NeverAgain movement. He spoke at rallies. He appeared on CNN, Fox, MSNBC, ABC, and CBS to make a forceful case for gun reform. After amassing a huge following on Twitter and becoming a political force to be reckoned with, Hogg used his new-found power and influence to force major organizations to change their ways. For example, he organized a "die-in" at Publix, a large supermarket chain that supported Republican gubernatorial candidate Adam Putnam over his staunch alliance with the NRA. Under public pressure, Publix announced that they would no longer support Putnam's candidacy. After becoming the target of online bullying by Fox News talk-show host Laura Ingraham, Hogg called for a boycott of her show, prompting 24 advertisers to pull their support. Ingraham was forced to issue an apology to Hogg and subsequently took a leave of absence.[22]

The March for Our Lives

Although the #NeverAgain campaign is still alive and well as of this writing, some eight months after the Parkland massacre, by far the pinnacle of the campaign was the historic March for Our Lives, held on March 24, 2018. The March for Our Lives attracted 1.2 million people, making it one of the largest youth protest events since the Vietnam War.[23] Conceived just four days after the Parkland massacre, the March for Our Lives unleashed a powerful rush of anger and frustration all over America—visceral emotions that had been building and bottling up for years, but which had never before been given such a prominent public outlet for their expression. The announcement for the event instantly attracted widespread and unwavering support, not just from young people all over the world but also from older generations. Dozens of high-profile celebrities declared their solidarity and support for the event, including Amal and George Clooney, Steven Spielberg, Alyssa Milano, John Legend, Paul McCartney, Jimmy Fallon, Will Smith, and Oprah Winfrey. The Clooneys, Spielberg, Oprah, and others collectively donated hundreds of millions of dollars to support the march.[24] Even President Barack Obama, who had been keeping a low profile since leaving office in 2017, broke his long silence to voice his support for the event. He tweeted, "Michelle and I are so inspired by all the young people who made today's marches happen. Keep at it. You're leading us forward. Nothing can stand in the way of millions of voices calling for change."[25] While the main event was held on Pennsylvania Avenue in Washington, D.C., dozens of parallel demonstrations were held all across the United States. In Boston, the local demonstration attracted 80,000 people.[26] In New York City, it attracted over 200,000 people.[27] Events were also held across Canada,[28] Europe, and even Asia.[29]

The main event at Washington featured most of the Parkland student leaders of the #NeverAgain movement. It also featured several survivors and the family members of victims from other major American school shootings. It featured Yolanda Renee King, granddaughter of Martin Luther King Jr., a notable victim of gun violence in America. The young King, only nine years old, told the audience, "My grandfather had a dream that his four little children will not be judged by the color of their skin, but by the content of their character." She went on to say, "I have a dream that enough is enough, and that this should be a gun-free world, period."[30]

But the undeniable highlight of the entire event was the powerful speech by Emma González. Dressed in her signature irreverent style—torn jeans, denim jacket covered with patches and buttons—González timed her speech to be the same length as the total time of the Parkland massacre. She interrupted her own speech with an eerie period of silence, during which she looked into the crowd, tears running down her face. After four minutes, a timer went off. González resumed speaking. "Since the time that I came out here," she said, "it has been 6 minutes and 20 seconds. The shooter has ceased shooting and will soon abandon his rifle, blend in with the students as they escape and walk free for an hour before arrest. Fight for your lives, before it's someone else's job."[31] Her powerful, haunting speech left her audience in tears. It was the most memorable moment of the entire event. As the *Washington Post* put it, González "moved a nation."[32]

Backlash and Response

The force of the #NeverAgain movement has been so powerful that reactionary conservatives have aggressively attacked, trolled, and threatened the Parkland survivors. One of the most vile attacks came from right-wing conspiracy theorists who claimed that the Parkland shooting victims and survivors were all "crisis actors," paid for by the liberal media and political establishment to create fear and panic and persuade Americans to give up their guns.[33] Leslie Gibson, a Republican candidate for Maine's House of Representatives, lashed out at Emma González, calling her a "skinhead lesbian." He similarly lashed out at David Hogg, calling him a "bald-faced liar."[34] Jamie Allman, host of a nightly radio show on KDNL in St. Louis, threatened to sodomize Hogg with a "hot poker."[35] Conservative rock musician Ted Nugent characterized the Parkland students as "soulless" liars.[36] Right-wing talking head Erick Erickson branded Hogg a "bully."[37] Conspiracy theorist Alex Jones, host of the notorious disinformation site InfoWars, claimed to be a victim of Hogg's bullying.[38]

But the most extreme attack came in the form of a call to law enforcement falsely reporting a hostage situation at the home of David Hogg.[39] Known as "swatting," this type of prank has been used by trolls looking either for a cheap laugh or to bully and harass innocent people.[40] The danger of swatting is that police arrive on the scene prepared for a tense situation and are therefore more likely to pull the trigger. Swatting has in the past resulted in death.[41] While it is unclear whether the swatting of Hogg's family was for mere amusement or to exact deadly revenge, the outcome could well have been fatal.

Yet, the Parkland students refused to be cowed and defeated by the threats, bullying, intimidation, and harassment by their critics. Instead they fought back, calling out the trolls online, even responding with humor. After the NRA released a video in which spokesperson Dana Loesch attacked the Parkland survivors and accused them of being part of a liberal plot to suppress freedom, Parkland student Sarah Chadwick released a parody video reproducing much of the content of the original but redirecting the outrage back at the NRA.[42] The parody video became a viral hit across social media. As Craig Silverman, media editor for Buzzfeed News, remarked, "They're kind of trolling the trolls back, and in some ways I think that might be pretty effective."[43]

According to other commentators, the Parkland students have indeed been effective, not just in pushing back against the trolls, but also in winning the culture war over guns in America. As Peter Beinart noted in *The Atlantic*, the effect of the Parkland students' activism has been profound.

At least 20 major corporations, including Hertz, United Airlines, and Metlife, have ended their partnerships with the NRA. Dick's Sporting Goods and Walmart have both decided they will no longer sell guns to people under the age of 21. Beinart also rightly noted that at a CNN town hall, Senator Marco Rubio and Dana Loesch were both put on the defensive following the sharp and forceful criticisms of the Parkland students, their parents, their teachers, and an angry audience.[44]

Indeed, seeing the #NeverAgain campaign through the broader lens of the culture wars is perhaps the most useful way of gauging the campaign's success. As Benjamin Hart observed in the *New York Magazine* (http:nymag. com), the Parkland teens managed to pull off the unthinkable. Republicans formerly wielded solid control of the public discourse over guns. But after Parkland, they lost all control of that discourse. That loss was not due solely to the horror of the Parkland massacre; rather, it had so much to do with the tireless and persistent campaign on the part the Parkland survivors to hammer this issue into the public conscience through repeated media appearances and social media activism.[45] Dylan Matthews from *Vox* noted that the Parkland students have managed to shift public opinion in measurable terms toward stronger support for gun control.[46] Indeed, according to a Gallup poll conducted just weeks after Parkland, public support for stricter gun laws reached its highest level since 1993, standing at a remarkable 67 percent.[47]

In terms of legal and institutional change, Florida, long known for its loose gun laws, responded to the Parkland students by raising the minimum age to purchase a gun to 21. It also introduced a waiting period as well as new measures enabling law enforcement to confiscate guns from individuals who pose a security risk.[48] But the most stunning effect of the #NeverAgain movement has been the serious toll inflicted upon the NRA. New York state governor Andrew Cuomo instructed the Department of Financial Services to look into all financial and insurance companies with ties to the NRA and to pressure them to cut those ties.[49] The move appears to have worked. In 2018, the NRA filed a lawsuit against the state of New York, claiming that the "blacklisting" campaign is driving the veteran gun-lobbying organization out of business.[50] According to the lawsuit, the NRA lost "tens of millions of dollars." It claims the NRA is in "deep financial trouble"[51] and may soon be "unable to exist."[52] While the Parkland students obviously did not direct the New York state DFS to pressure the banking and insurance industry to cut their ties to the NRA, they *did* create the cultural conditions under which such a move could even be conceivable. Indeed, the DFS justified this move by citing "increasing public backlash against the NRA and like organizations."[53]

Thus, it turns out, the impassioned speeches, the television interviews, the talk show appearances, the social media campaigns, the boycotts, and the historic March for Our Lives all brought about a seismic shift in the culture wars that sparked an institutional response. To put the matter bluntly, the Parkland students achieved what decades of gun control activism by previous generations had failed to achieve: shifting the cultural tide against the American love affair with guns.

The Kids Are All Right

My aim in this chapter is not to critique technological determinism per se but rather to critique a popular narrative that conveniently shields the political economic order from critical scrutiny and directs public outrage and anxiety at teenagers and technology—technology, not as driven by political and economic forces, but rather technology as possessing magical powers of seduction, which charm and entice only the weak and the naive. The ideal targets of blame, according to the current popular framing of technology, are young people for having allowed themselves to be seduced by technology. This seduction narrative of smartphones and social media requires a conception of the teenage subject as essentially a powerless, uncritical, and passive simpleton, utterly bereft of will and agency. It paints a pathetic picture of teenagers as pitiful creatures so badly lacking in self-discipline, drive, determination, and personality that they almost demand a judgment of contempt. The seduction narrative, by design, forces the conclusion that teenagers have only themselves to blame.

Herein lies the problem with the seduction narrative: it fits squarely within a neoliberal worldview, which envisions a social universe inhabited by so many autonomous individuals, each responsible for his or her own fate. According to this worldview, we need not pay attention to larger systems and structures, for there are no structural reasons for social problems. There are only patterns among autonomous individuals. Thus, if teenagers really are depressed, antisocial, hypersensitive, fragile, lazy, incompetent, and on and on and on, that's on them, not on the larger political economic system of which they happen to be a part. If they cannot afford college tuition fees, if they cannot find a job, if they have no hope or prospect of moving out of their parents' homes and starting a life of their own, then it's entirely their fault for having wasted their time and having rotted their minds in front of a smartphone screen.

The fallacy of the seduction narrative of technology is not only that it paints a false picture of teenagers but also that it feeds a culture of condescension toward them. After Parkland, the persistence of such condescension—the enduring belief that the opinions of teenagers don't matter, because they are hopelessly lost in virtual worlds online and too antisocial and immature to participate in political discourse to say anything that matters—is dangerous and irresponsible. The #NeverAgain movement, I wish to argue, completely undermines the narrative of Millennial laziness and incompetence, as well as the seduction narrative of technology. The Parkland students, and the millions of young people they inspired, pulled off a historic feat that completely defies the picture painted by LA Reel House Media's "A Millennial Job Interview" and Jean Twenge's "Have Smart Phones Destroyed A Generation?" The #Never-Again movement demonstrated the exceptional maturity, political intelligence, cultural awareness, technological adeptness, and fierce, resolute determination of young people to create a different word for themselves and those who come after.

It also demonstrates the power of social media to bring about a cultural revolution. Technology has indeed changed our culture—but not in the way that the seduction narrative or anti-Millennial rhetoric imagines. Social media have changed the terrain of public discourse, enabling both destructive, antisocial trolling and constructive political organizing. The vicious personal attacks against the Parkland students by adult media personalities reveals that it's *not* young people who have been adversely shaped by technology but rather the adults. On the contrary, the Parkland students showed that they understand the new terrain, that they know how to navigate it and to harness its powers for a just cause. In this, they demonstrated, not mindless passivity, but rather critically engaged political agency. In short, they showed that it's the adults who have a problem and that the kids are all right.

Notes

1. LA Reel House Media, "A Millennial Job Interview," October 24, 2017, https://www.youtube.com/watch?v=Uo0KjdDJr1c.

2. For more examples of anti-Millennial rhetoric, see Bruce Tulgan, *Not Everyone Gets a Trophy: How to Manage the Millennials* (New York: John Wiley & Sons, 2016); Jean M. Twenge, *Generation Me—Revised and Updated: Why Today's Young Americans Are More Confident, Assertive, Entitled—and More Miserable Than Ever Before* (New York: Atria, 2006); Joel Stein, "Millennials: The Me Me Me Generation," *Time*, May 20, 2013, http://time.com/247/millennials-the-me-me-me-generation/; Kathy Buckworth, "Millennials Need to Change These 5 Attitudes about Work," *HuffPost*, March 24, 2016, https://www.huffingtonpost.ca/kathy-buckworth/millennial-attitudes_b_9538754.html.

3. For commentary on this phenomenon, see Sophia A. McClennen, "How Pervasive Anti-Millennial Sentiment Has Hurt the Cause of Student Protesters," *Conversation*, December 4, 2015, https://theconversation.com/how-pervasive -anti-millennial-sentiment-has-hurt-the-cause-of-student-protesters-51234; Eleanor Robertson, "Why Are the Baby Boomers Desperate to Make Millennials Hate Ourselves?" *Guardian*, September 4, 2015, https://www.theguardian.com /commentisfree/2015/sep/04/why-are-the-baby-boomers-desperate-to-make-us -millennials-hate-ourselves.

4. Jean Twenge, "Have Smart Phones Destroyed a Generation?" *Atlantic*, September 2017, https://www.theatlantic.com/magazine/archive/2017/09/has-the-smart phone-destroyed-a-generation/534198/.

5. Ibid.

6. For commentary on this aspect of Marx's thought, see Andrew Feenberg, "The Ambivalence of Technology," *Sociological Perspectives* 33, no. 1 (1990): 35–50.

7. Harold Innis, *The Bias of Communication* (Toronto, ON: University of Toronto Press, 1951).

8. Marshall McLuhan, *Understanding Media: The Extensions of Man* (Cambridge, MA: MIT Press, 1994), Chapter 1.

9. Neil Postman, *Amusing Ourselves to Death: Public Discourse in the Age of Show Business* (New York: Penguin, 2006).

10. See Andrew Feenberg, *Critical Theory of Technology* (Oxford: Oxford University Press, 1991); *Questioning Technology* (London: Routledge, 1991); *Transforming Technology* (Oxford: Oxford University Press, 2002); Douglas Kellner, "Multiple Literacies and Critical Pedagogy in a Multicultural Society," *Educational Theory* 48, no. 1 (1998): 103–22; "Technological Transformation, Multiple Literacies, and the Re-Visioning of Education," *E-Learning and Digital Media* 1, no. 1 (2004): 9–37; Douglas Kellner and Jeff Share, "Toward Critical Media Literacy: Core Concepts, Debates, Organizations, and Policy," *Discourse: Studies in the Cultural Politics of Education* 26, no. 3 (2005): 369–86.

11. Oliver Laughland, Richard Luscombe, and Alan Yuhas, "Florida School Shooting: At Least 17 People Dead on 'Horrific, Horrific Day,'" *Guardian*, February 15, 2018, https://www.theguardian.com/us-news/2018/feb/14/florida-shoot ing-school-latest-news-stoneman-douglas.

12. Ray Sanchez, "Florida School Shooter Nikolas Cruz Indicted on 34 Counts, Including Premeditated Murder," *CNN*, March 7, 2018, https://www .cnn.com/2018/03/07/us/nikolas-cruz-indictment/index.html.

13. Emily Witt, "How the Survivors of Parkland Began the Never Again Movement," *New Yorker*, February 19, 2018, https://www.newyorker.com/news/news -desk/how-the-survivors-of-parkland-began-the-never-again-movement.

14. Valerie Strauss, "This Parkland Student Quickly Amassed More Twitter Followers Than the NRA. Here's What She's Been Writing," *Washington Post*, March 1, 2018, https://www.washingtonpost.com/news/answer-sheet/wp/2018 /03/01/this-parkland-student-quickly-amassed-more-twitter-followers-than -the-nra-heres-what-shes-been-writing/.

15. CNN Staff, "Florida Student Emma Gonzalez to Lawmakers and Gun Advocates: 'We Call BS,'" *CNN*, February 17, 2018, https://www.cnn.com/2018 /02/17/us/florida-student-emma-gonzalez-speech/index.html.

16. Ibid.

17. Delaney Tarr, "I Survived the Parkland Shooting. This Is What I Want Everyone to Know," *Teen Vogue*, February 19, 2018, https://www.teenvogue.com /story/i-survived-the-parkland-shooting-delaney-tarr.

18. Ibid.

19. Cameron Kasky, "Parkland Student: My Generation Won't Stand for This," *CNN*, February 20, 2018, https://www.cnn.com/2018/02/15/opinions/florida -shooting-no-more-opinion-kasky/index.html.

20. Ibid.

21. Taylor Swaak, "Who Is Alfonso Calderon? Florida Shooting Survivor Gives Passionate Speech in Tallahassee," *Newsweek*, February 21, 2018, https://www .newsweek.com/who-alfonso-calderon-815220.

22. Kyle Arnold, Paul Brinkmann, and Mark Skoneki, "Publix Suspends Political Contributions as David Hogg 'Die-ins' Begin," *Orlando Sentinel*, May 25, 2018, https://www.orlandosentinel.com/business/os-orlando-publix-die-in-2018 0525-story.html.

23. German Lopez, "It's Official: March for Our Lives Was One of the Biggest Youth Protests since the Vietnam War," *Vox*, March 26, 2018, https://www.vox .com/policy-and-/2018/3/26/17160646/march-for-our-lives-crowd-size-count.

24. Christian Allaire, "All the Celebrities Who Showed Up for the March for Our Lives," *Vogue*, March 24, 2018. https://www.vogue.com/article/celebrities -march-for-our-lives-gun-violence-protest

25. Avery Anapol, "Obama Tweets Message of Support to 'March for Our Lives' participants," *Hill*, March 24, 2018, https://thehill.com/blogs/blog-briefing -room/380092-obama-tweets-message-of-support-to-march-for-our-lives-par ticipants.

26. WGBH News Staff, "Boston 'March For Our Lives' Organizers: We're Not Done Yet," *WGBH News*, March 26, 2018, https://www.wgbh.org/news /2018/03/26/local-news/boston-march-our-lives-organizers-were-not-done-yet.

27. Alan Judd , Vanessa McCray, Arlinda Smith Broady, and Tamar Hallerman, "In Atlanta and Across the Nation, Protesters Say, 'Enough Is Enough,'" *Atlanta Journal-Constitution*, March 24, 2018, https://www.myajc.com/news/atlanta-and -across-the-nation-protesters-say-enough-enough/M7A7E6mV44TPi9w7MM YVWO/.

28. The Canadian Press, "Canadian Cities Hold March for Our Lives Events," *CTV News,* March 24, 2018, https://www.ctvnews.ca/canada/canadian-cities -hold-march-for-our-lives-events-1.3857087.

29. Dakin Andone, Amanda Jackson, and Isabella Gomez, "The March for Our Lives Isn't Just Happening in the United States," *CNN*, March 24, 2018, https://www.cnn.com/2018/03/24/world/march-for-our-lives-around-the-world -trnd/index.html.

30. Jennifer Calfas, "'I Have a Dream That Enough Is Enough.' Martin Luther King Jr.'s Granddaughter, 9, Gives Powerful Speech at March For Our Lives," March 24, 2018, http://time.com/5214244/yolanda-renee-king-martin-luther-king-march-for-our-lives/.

31. Katie Reilly, "Emma González Kept America in Stunned Silence to Show How Quickly 17 People Died at Parkland," *Time*, March 24, 2018, http://time.com/5214322/emma-gonzalez-march-for-our-lives-speech/.

32. Peter Marks, "Emma González and the Wordless Act That Moved a Nation," *Washington Post*, March 25, 2018, https://www.washingtonpost.com/news/arts-and-entertainment/wp/2018/03/25/emma-gonzalez-and-the-wordless-act-that-moved-a-nation/.

33. Jason Wilson, "Crisis Actors, Deep State, False Flag: The Rise of Conspiracy Theory Code Words," *Guardian*, February 21, 2018, https://www.theguardian.com/us-news/2018/feb/21/crisis-actors-deep-state-false-flag-the-rise-of-conspiracy-theory-code-words.

34. Matt Stevens, "'Skinhead Lesbian' Tweet about Parkland Student Ends Maine Republican's Candidacy," *New York Times*, March 18, 2018, https://www.nytimes.com/2018/03/18/us/politics/maine-republican-leslie-gibson.html.

35. Eliot C. McLaughlin, "Sinclair TV Host Resigns after Making Vulgar Comment about Parkland Student David Hogg," *CNN*, April 10, 2018, https://www.cnn.com/2018/04/10/us/sinclair-commentator-resigns-jamie-allman-david-hogg/index.html.

36. Alessia Grunberger, "Ted Nugent Calls Parkland Survivors 'Liars' and 'Soulless' in Interview," *CNN*, April 2, 2018, https://www.cnn.com/2018/03/31/politics/nra-member-calls-parkland-survivors-liars/index.html.

37. Joe Difazio, "Conservative Commentator Erick Erickson Calls Parkland Shooting Survivor David Hogg 'A Bully,'" *Newsweek*, February 26, 2018, https://www.newsweek.com/david-hogg-nra-gun-rights-fox-news-florida-marjory-stoneman-douglas-high-821374

38. Madison Malone Kircher, "Alex Jones Says He's Being Bullied by a Teenage Stoneman-Shooting Survivor," *New York*, February 27, 2018, http://nymag.com/intelligencer/2018/02/alex-jones-says-hes-being-bullied-by-stonemans-david-hogg.html.

39. Richard Luscombe, "Florida School Shooting Survivor Targeted in 'Swatting' Prank," *Guardian*, June 5, 2018, https://www.theguardian.com/us-news/2018/jun/05/florida-school-shooting-survivor-david-hogg-swatting-v-prank.

40. Jason Fagone, "The Serial Swatter," *New York Times*, November 24, 2015, https://www.nytimes.com/2015/11/29/magazine/the-serial-swatter.html.

41. Benjamin Kentish, "British Man Charged after US Gamer Is Shot by Swat Police Following Hoax Terrorism Call," *Independent*, April 10, 2017, https://www.independent.co.uk/news/uk/home-news/robert-mcdaid-charged-tyran-dobbs-swatting-hoax-call-swat-terrorism-maryland-shot-gun-explosives-a7677071.html.

42. Brett Clarkson, "Parkland Student Sarah Chadwick Spoofs That Ominous NRA Ad," *Sun-Sentinel*, March 9, 2018, http://www.sun-sentinel.com/local/bro ward/parkland/florida-school-shooting/fl-reg-msd-sarah-chadwick-nra -20180308-story.html.

43. CBC Radio, "'They're Trolling the Trolls Back': How Parkland Survivors Are Responding to Conspiracy Theorists," February 23, 2018, https://www.cbc .ca/radio/day6/episode-378-school-shooting-conspiracies-olympic-stadiums -rip-arthur-black-a-i-jobs-martin-amis-and-more-1.4546905/they-re-trolling -the-trolls-back-how-parkland-survivors-are-responding-to-conspiracy-the orists-1.4546938.

44. Peter Beinart, "Conservatives Are Losing the Culture War over Guns," *Atlantic*, March 1, 2018, https://www.theatlantic.com/politics/archive/2018/03 /conservatives-are-losing-the-culture-war-over-guns/554585/.

45. Benjamin Hart, "The Parkland Teens Are Winning the Culture War," *New York*, March 31, 2018, http://nymag.com/intelligencer/2018/03/the-parkland -teens-are-winning-the-culture-war.html?

46. Dylan Matthews, "More Americans Say Guns Are the Country's Top Issue Than Ever Have Before," *Vox*, March 9, 2018, https://www.vox.com /2018/3/29/17157468/parkland-shooting-public-opinion-gun-control-gun-law -polling.

47. Jeffrey Jones, "U.S. Preference for Stricter Gun Laws Highest Since 1993," *Gallup*, March 14, 2018, https://news.gallup.com/poll/229562/preference-stricter -gun-laws-highest-1993.aspx.

48. Athena Jones, Darran Simon, and Carolyn Sung, "Florida Senate OKs Bill Raising Age to Buy Guns, Banning Bump Stock Sales," *CNN*, March 5, 2018, https://www.cnn.com/2018/03/05/us/urgent-gun-measures-florida-state-legisla tures/index.html.

49. Matt Ford, "Andrew Cuomo's Trumpian War on the NRA," *New Republic*, August 28, 2018, https://newrepublic.com/article/150933/andrew-cuomos-trum pian-war-nra.

50. Jon Schuppe, "NRA Says New York 'Blacklisting Campaign' Is Driving It Out of Business," *NBC News*, August 3, 2018, https://www.nbcnews.com/news /us-news/nra-says-new-york-blacklisting-campaign-driving-it-out-business -n897521.

51. Emily Price, "NRA Claims 'Deep Financial Trouble' May Soon Put It Out of Business," *Fortune*, August 3, 2018, http://fortune.com/2018/08/03/nra -claims-deep-financial-trouble-may-put-it-out-of-business/.

52. Ewan Palmer, "Is the NRA Going Bankrupt? Group Claims It Will Soon Be 'Unable to Exist' Due to Financial Difficulties," *Newsweek*, August 4, 2018, https://www.newsweek.com/nra-going-bankrupt-group-claim-it-will-soon -be-unable-exist-due-financial-1057187.

53. New York Department of Financial Services, Memorandum, April 19, 2018, https://www.dfs.ny.gov/legal/dfs/DFS_Guidance_Risk_Management_NRA _Gun_Manufacturers-Insurance.pdf.

CHAPTER NINE

Anonymity and (Mis)representation on Social Media Are Changing Who We Are and How We Think About Identity

Jessica Lowell Mason

Just as water, gas, and electricity are brought into our houses from far off to satisfy our needs in response to a minimal effort, so shall we be supplied with visual and auditory images, which will appear and disappear at the simple movement of the hand, hardly more than a sign. . . . I don't know if a philosopher has ever dreamed of a company engaged in the home delivery of Sensory Reality.

Paul Valery, "The Conquest of Ubiquity"[1]

How we see ourselves and others is changing as we become more dependent on technology. Social media does not simply offer new ways to connect with one another; it offers new ways to represent ourselves and develop our identities. This affects our self-concepts and concept of reality. With the proliferation of bots on Twitter, fake accounts on Face-book, role-playing venues such as Second Life, and other platforms for cyber representation, our cyber-, flesh-, and cognitive identities are simul-taneously conflating and splintering. We now face the prospect of going beyond our former identity concepts. But what questions do advances in cyber representation raise about who we are and the way we think and process information when our ability to manipulate information is imbri-cated with our inability to control it?

Our Cyberized Lives, Our Natural Deaths

Lewis Carroll's whimsical and absurdist tale, *Alice's Adventures in Won-derland*, begins with a small child at the precipice of the imagination, an imagination that might be said to belong to her alone but that challenges us to question both that assertion and reality itself. Boredom, curiosity, and a demand for pictures and conversations to occupy a restless state of mind propel young Alice from a flash of contemplation to the hurried, harried rabbit of impatience, which leads her to leap without a thought "down the rabbit hole" of the imagination. This deep well, this abyss of sorts, transports Alice into queer situations in which the paradigms of traditional logic no longer apply.

During the course of her queer adventures, Alice's understanding of language shifts, and she becomes a carrier for a new consciousness; she shrinks, she grows, she finds herself in precarious situations with unfa-miliar figures, ones that require alternative forms of sense-making. The entire cacophony of meaning that defines Alice's adventures are perception-altering, reality-distorting, hallucinogenic, sometimes danger-ous, often absurd, and rife with juxtapositions and paradoxes that serve as the new norms for navigating the world and relationality. Yet, though this plethora of peculiarity constitutes a new life of the mind, it is simultane-ously a location of death: the death of reality as we know it, which must accompany the birth of an alternate reality. The wild adventures of Alice, which appeared in 1865, make up a strangely accurate premonition of the wondrous and catastrophic impact that technological advances have had and are having on consciousness and identity in the 21st century.

In many ways, we have entered a twilight zone of terrific and terrible technology that is both in and out of our grasp. We are in the throes of an age defined by surreality, self-deception, and social media, all of which, in some contexts, can be treated as exchangeable synonyms, but each of which should be interrogated independently. Like Alice, we have cata-pulted ourselves into an abyss constituted by marvels and dangers we never could have anticipated. Our sense is that it is from our own imaginations that we have created a world over which we perceive ourselves as having control when in fact we have very little control, but our imaginations are not insular—they are influenced by outside forces, including the political and institutional contexts within which social media technologies were developed. It is as Mary Shelley predicted: we are a scientific species without wisdom, a Frankenstein nation, giving birth to that which we are not prepared to oversee. We manage to give birth to technological creatures, to social media monsters, but we do so without the ability to predict outcomes, domino effects, full pictures, and the ways our world and our identities will be irreparably altered. Social media, an industry run for corporate profit, calls on us to follow its manic applications into a black hole of social consciousness, and we, startled and entranced by the intensity and chaos, throw ourselves into it.

A thousand metaphors for the effects of social media technologies upon our lives would not even scratch the surface of the transformative deluge into which we have entered and are now perambulating. Our new and altered social media reality is reshaping the way we think and who we are, and, despite how dangerous this could be to our health and survival, we most often barely give this a thought as we plunge into dimensions unknown in a world that we have created and that has been created for us. We are living new cyberized lives, but at what cost? What, of our humanity, are we losing as we dive deeper and deeper into this rabbit hole of cyber-altered consciousness?

Pins, Pints, and Pining: Postconsumerism and the Consumption of Identity

What we once might have considered "singular" metaphorical identities have now become conglomerates of virtual identity: fractured, distorted, reconstituted, and multiplied by social media platforms, such as Facebook, Twitter, Snapchat, Instagram, Reddit, Tumblr, Google+, MySpace, LinkedIn, and Pinterest. Each one of these platforms for the dissemination and mobilization of identity has its own distinct way of shattering and reconstituting selfhood, and these ways should interest and concern us. They provide opportunities for us to reject our inclination toward passivity, even as they make it easier and easier for us to take a passive role. By concerning ourselves with the effect of social media on identity, and by exercising critical and analytic thought on our virtual representation practices, we might be able to develop new agency, which could empower us to influence both the technologies themselves and our uses of them.

First, we should consider this loaded question: What is a virtual identity, and are all identities, in some sense, virtual? In the sense that identity is a combinatory and symbolic construction with material consequences, yes, identity is always partly virtual. It is both virtual and material, conceptual and concrete, relating to cognition and relating to cultural practice. Given that identity itself always already possesses a degree of virtuality, the addition of social media identity virtuality renders identity doubly virtual. To refer to a "virtual identity" is, then, to refer to a virtualized already virtual concept.

Updates in social media technologies have ushered in changes and new insights, but they also have placed new limitations on insight, to our self-concepts, our material experiences of identity, and our psychic experiences of selfhood, as well as to our categorizations of identity. Consider a benign example of an identity-altering social media platform: the virtual and virtually endless bulletin board known as Pinterest. Pinterest is a web application company some would consider to be more on the periphery of social media than other similar media platforms because, on the surface, it appears to be an organizational device; however, the information- and image-hoarding application is not immune to the identity-constructing (and -deconstructing) practices of its virtual contemporaries. Pinterest, with millions of active users, is one piece in a quickly evolving and always changing puzzle of social media technology. In this global matrix of virtual representation, the company cannot distance itself from the role it plays; despite its creators' attempts to emphasize its storage features and separate it from other social media sites, giving it a more educational and purposeful feel, the site's function makes obvious its social component. Though Pinterest classifies itself as a tool for visual discovery, collection, and storage, with the primary aim of encouraging its users to use discovery as a platform for physical actions, such as might be implied by the prevalence of food/recipe-related DIY (do-it-yourself) pins on the site, this only accounts for a portion of the site's content.

The notion of Pinterest as purely a storage tool fails to take into account its social dimension and the space it provides for identity construction, both of which are foundational to the platform and evidenced in its applied uses. Pinterest users are not just hoarding images and information; there is much more to it than that—they are inserting their preferences and their identities into a social sphere of representation. To pin up an image of a meal that one wants to make in the future or that one wishes she were consuming at the present moment is not merely to catalog information— not when the momentary act of seeing an image becomes a social act of memorialization and preservation on a social media platform. When an individual transitions from a moment of desired or planned consumption (e.g., wanting the food porn cherry pie pictured, wishing for the staged bedroom photographed, lusting after that pint of Butter Beer gelato repinned across hundreds of Harry Potter–themed boards, planning to buy the plum cashmere cloak hanging over the model in the photograph) to a moment of preservation, he or she is doing so using a platform that is inherently social and that involves representation. The act of pinning on Pinterest is a social act, not a utilitarian one. The pinner engages in the public spectacle of virtual consumerism without necessarily having to be a consumer: he or she wants and likes but does not necessarily buy—and there is no system in place to determine her intentions when she engages in pinning, so it is all mixed into the muddle of virtual social and consumer ambiguity, where the lines between consumption, representation, and identity are crossed and where these dimensions of social media technology are blurred. In this way, Pinterest, like its sibling social media sites, plays on our need to represent our identities and fuses this need with materialism.

Any critical inquiry into the functionality and consequences of Pinterest on our individual and collective lives must always resist the temptation to give in to our consumerist impulses. While some pinners may use Pinterest as a private storage device, many do not. A large portion, and perhaps a majority, of Pinterest users are using the site more as a platform for social connection and consumerist representation than as a practical matter of private storage. Pinterest's consumerist component is entangled with its function as a social platform. And employees of the site want this to continue, for there would be no Pinterest without the pairing of imagistic virtual identity construction with consumerist impulses and market consequences.

There is no virtual identity construction without the social components of seeing and being seen. Pinterest, like many of its sister sites, is all about visuality in the form of collective voyeurism and exhibition, virtual engagement, and the evasion of physical obligation—we are not consuming, we are merely virtually consuming; our minds, not our bodies, are consuming, and we are doing this through the social media paradox of virtual collective action, alone-and-together. Look no further than the basic components of the site itself for evidence of Pinterest's social media import: as on many other web application sites, such as Twitter and Instagram, each Pinterest user can follow other users and can also be followed. In addition, each user has profile features through which he or she can represent and describe his or her "self" in a limited number of characters via a minibiography, to display a photographic representation of him- or herself, and to shape in a modest way the aesthetic representation of that self via the profile. The personalization features of Pinterest include the ability to name and write a short description for each virtual board on which virtual pins will be stored and shared. A user might label a gothic/literary-themed Pinterest board "Everything Poe-tic" and then proceed to write a cryptic description of his or her individual interpretation of the images (words, art, videos, etc.) that constitute the board. The site is predicated on the concept of sharing—idea sharing, but this idea sharing is imbued with identity representation: users show *who they are* through the images they pin up on the board. Pins may be shared, and boards may be shared, but this results in a transformation of personal ownership and challenges our notion of identity as fixed and pertaining to a singular self. If a user makes a demonstration of his or her identity (who he or she is) through a board that another user follows, the follower of the board is making a public social statement of identification with that user and with the perspective or philosophy of identity that the board is promoting. The identity, as expressed by the pins, is commodified because many of the pins are produced by companies selling products and trying to get users to click on the pins in order to be transported to their websites.

Our Pinterest boards and our pins certainly represent us, and we come to identify with them, and the virtual social storage medium itself encourages this. It does so by making pin-sharing incredibly easy and by not requiring that sources be identified or linked to any fixed entity. One does not necessarily know where a pin came from when one repins it. In order to "create" a pin, one does not have to actually have created the image or the object featured in the image, and neither does one have to identify or attach a source to a pin—one has the ability to pin, or project, an image onto a board without context or of framing it in an invented context, a context one makes up or one set by the invented theme of the board. The titles given to users and their boards place the virtual materiality of the consumerist images into a framework of personal identification, a framework that each user has the ability to construct but one that is also inherently shaped by already existing images and virtual consumerist culture. Pinterest is not an example of postconsumerism in a postapocalyptic sense; it is an example of postconsumerism in a literal sense: users are *posting* virtual representations of their consumerism and forming and establishing identities that are imbedded within that consumerism. Our self-concepts are being consumed by virtual consumerism: proverbially eaten up, digested, and spit out by technologies that are commodifying consciousness. We are investing in our images, in images that represent our identities, and the corporate platforms through which we're doing it are investing in our psychic dependency on materialist representation. As our ineffable identities are becoming corporately virtualized, our virtual identities are becoming commodities. This means that we are being reprogrammed psychically by our social media technologies to consume that which the technologies tell us we should buy, and largely under the not-entirely-true belief that we, not our social media accounts, are in control. Rather than following Descartes's philosophy—"I think, therefore I am"—we practicing the new consumerist philosophy of "I buy, therefore I am"—or "I *intend* to buy, therefore I am. It is not that we are without agency; it is that our agency is being delivered to us by social media companies that encourage us to believe we are expressing who we are when, in fact, we are responding to products. Are we representing our "selves" or misrepresenting ourselves when we become part of the virtual machine of commodity? When what we "like" and what we share become outward manifestations of our inner consciousness (who we are), how do we know when we've crossed the line between autonomy and automation?

Consumerist objects are represented on Pinterest in often highly orchestrated and carefully devised pop-culture images, such as those featuring fashion models donning designer apparel and aesthetically pleasing color-popping photos of food taken by food photographers for food magazines. To repin is to announce one's identification with a representation of materiality. It must also be noted that the form of photographic representation that constitutes the "pin" is a copy—or a copy of a copy of a copy. Add to that the nature of repinning itself, which is to replicate a copy that is treated as an original but that is never actually an original because it is always a photograph, always a representation, always a virtual fragment of reality made virtually material. To pin is to represent a desire for something or a desire to be seen *as something* by others. Pinterest involves both subtle and profound acts of identification and self-representation—the abundance of art-themed boards makes this clear. Pinners may hoard photographic representations of art, their own art or artwork by others, organizing their preferences by creating boards according to either the names of their artists of preference or by themes that they feel are present in the works of a variety of artists—the organizational possibilities are endless, but it is obvious that organization, in this case, is a form of identification and representation.

Just as an interior designer might set up a room with art and books in order to represent a mood and style evocative of the person or family inhabiting that space, Pinterest boards serve as virtual personal spaces for "interior design" (identity construction) and representation. For a person to pin an art piece he or she detests without at least funneling it into a board labeled "Art I Detest" would be an unlikely act, almost as unlikely as it would be for a person who practices Judaism to post a pinned image of a C. S. Lewis quote hanging over the faded off-white robes of a depiction of Jesus. Pins and boards, the virtual galleries that Pinterest provides, represent identities and identifications, and they do so in a social way: the identities we depict via public image storage are shared identities. Whether or not Pinterest promotes itself as a space for the construction and dissemination of identity, the interaction between the application and its users, or the "lived virtual experience" of its users, makes obvious the fact that it is a medium for technoself formation and representation.

The Material Productions of Mistaken Identities: Social Media and the Cloning of Selfhood

Issues of identity and representation have been around since long before the proliferation of social media technologies. The effects of social media on identity require that new forms of cultural critique be performed; we need to broach the subject of the commodification of identity by social media companies and examine the role we play in this commodification, as well as how we are affected psychically by it. There is no question as to whether or not social media corporations are invested in and play a role in the exchange of cultural capital as it is influenced by the assertion of identity. There are profits to be made where identities are reified, and now, thanks to the popularity of social media, reification is a virtual process offering companies virtually limitless ways to profit off of our fragmented virtual assertions of selfhood. Images are integral to this process. The technical mass (re)production of images on social media sites, such as Facebook, Pinterest, and Twitter, is resulting in a surplus of commoditized representative and misrepresentative identity markers, and this raises questions related to authenticity and originality. These identity markers are images that we create through technology that dictates to us what we should create and that encourages us to become producers in the social media economy by producing images of ourselves and what we like. Who we are, and what we are, are virtual products to social media companies; this is why, when individuals write blogs and become popular enough among other users, social media companies offer them income in exchange for being able to place ads on their sites: being seen by more people is equal to an advertising opportunity in this context, and the construction of virtual identity is, therefore, profitable, so the technology continues to develop and encourage identity making in order to increase its profit margins. Sites encourage us to show more and more of ourselves, creating an identity surplus. Is this surplus in the virtual production of images of selfhood causing a disruption in our authenticity, a barrier against the formation of our identities, or is it moving us closer to our "ideal selves"? Both may be happening. An ideal self can exist without a tangible connection to a real, or authentic, self, and under the influence of social media, it is becoming harder and harder to distinguish between the two; however, "ideal" implies a perfection that we are incapable of achieving in reality: we may not become the ideal representation of our self, which is made ideal by virtue of its preservation and detachment from the real, but the technologies we use allow us to feed the fantasy that we might.

We cannot become the photo, we cannot become the selfie—we can only create the selfie and continue to be ourselves. But what happens when we, collectively, become fixated so much on these ideal selves, our artistic representations and the lives they live together and apart from us in virtual reality, that we neglect or become dissociated from our real selves, indescribable as they are? When one promotes images on social media of an "ideal self," the self that is made ideal only through the preservational (mis)representation of itself, one runs the risk of being so focused on constructing and managing this not-entirely-representative ideal that one shortchanges the development and nurturance of one's authentic self. Authenticity cannot be measured, but it is possible to consider inauthenticity in order to understand authenticity. Social media companies might encourage us to be less than honest with one another— but this is no different than most other avenues in our lives would do the same. For the purpose of this essay, authenticity is meant to mean honesty. An authentic self is an honest one. If one promotes an idealized version of oneself that does not accurately represent who one is in other areas of one's life, then one is being inauthentic—or dishonest. The question of whether or not social media encourages us to be honest or dishonest is important to ask, but social media cannot be held responsible for making liars; it can, however, be questioned regarding the way it gives power and a platform to liars. The idealization of the self is something that social media feeds into, not exactly as an overt promotion of narcissism but as an expression of our link to the ineffable; it is this fixation with the constant reproduction of idealizing representations of selfhood that virtual technologies promote and that social media companies exploit.

Our questions and concerns today over the ways social media technology is changing the way we understand identity mirror the questions and concerns raised by Walter Benjamin in his 1936 essay, "The Work of Art in the Age of Mechanical Reproduction."[2] Mechanical reproduction has exploded in the 21st century; the virtual reproduction of images on social media platforms is now the norm, and the reproduction and mass sharing of image reproductions has multiplied well beyond anything that existed in the 20th century. But the questions and concerns remain. How do we understand identity when identity and art are both conflating and dividing before our eyes but out of reach of our existing paradigms? One of Benjamin's observations about artistic reproduction is that it lacks something that the object of reproduction possesses. "Even the most perfect reproduction of work," he asserts, "is lacking in one element: its presence in time and space, its unique existence at the place where it happens to be".[3] Benjamin's observation, which supports the idea that photography creates room for us to reframe this lack in positive terms, is one that can be applied and understood where social media selfhood is concerned. Social media production of "work" does not attempt perfection in the sense that it has taken the goal of perfection, in most regards, out of the virtual reproduction equation, despite its goal of idealization of the self. This is the paradox of social media reproduction: the ideal itself is an ideal of distortion.

The reproductive idealization of selfhood on social media it not the idealization of authenticity; it is the *virtual* idealization of a *virtual* self, a self that is constructed and devised, one that is meant to reflect a fragmented piece in the narrative puzzle of selfhood about an authentic object but not an exact replication of the object. The goal of virtual reproduction is less to replicate than to refract, enhance, distort, or exaggerate. This is why the Facebook Messenger app allows users to virtually alter their "selves" according to their wishes (which are dictated and limited by the available options). This is why it allows for our eyeballs to be enlarged, for flames to line the lids of our eyes, for sparks to fly from our faces, for fire to burst out of our mouths when we open them, for koala bear ears and bamboo leaf crowns to sit atop our heads, for red rose petals to fall down over our heads as our cheeks are rouged to match an imposed pink surrounding, and for animated versions of our selves to coexist, through the application's mirror of distortion, with our living flesh-and-blood selves. This is why filters on Instagram allow users to adjust the color and lighting of their images before sharing, and why the hashtags #filter and #nofilter exist. This is why selfie-taking apps like Pics Art allow users to choose from effects, such as Magic, Blur, Artistic, Pop Art, Paper, Distort, and Color, each of which has subeffects from which to choose. The Magic effect alone offers 35 different options, including but not limited to Flora,

Pastel, Undead, White Ice, Feast, Rainbow, Galaxy, Soul, Dystopia, Wonderland, and Money. What does it mean to distort (or enhance) one's reproduction by Money-ing it, or making it Moneid? Is it to represent selfhood? To distort it? To deconstruct it? To reproduce it? To alter the virtual self with the goal of stating a philosophical truth or making a political statement about the authentic self? Or is it to make virtual art of the actual self? It may be all of these things, and more. We need to begin asking ourselves what thought we are putting into acts of social media identity construction, such as the act of taking a selfie. Questioning our social media behavior may not seem relevant to some users, but there is much value in doing so to the average technologically savvy and to the pop-culture-critical individual alike. But for those who care to understand what we're doing, why we're doing it, and what it means for our future, asking such questions is of enormous value.

The authenticity that Benjamin claims relies upon "the presence of the original" is dismantled by the virtual reality of social media technology. While we might attempt to capture and share our authentic selves on social media in some instances, in others we might just as deliberately attempt to miscapture or misrepresent them. We might also attempt to capture, preserve, or represent the presence of our original selves in a given moment, but in the process of doing this, we might inadvertently create a version of our selves that is radically at odds with the self with which we most deeply identify. Virtual production allows us to be multiple selves or to be many versions of the same self or to deconstruct selfhood altogether. It has exploded our concepts of selfhood, originality, and authenticity, and distanced us from the internalization of these concepts. The explosions of these concepts is not necessarily negative, but it can be if we are not discerning—the distance social media has created in us from the internalization of the concept is problematic. We need more introspection if we are to move forward as thinking agents.

There are both positives and negatives associated with the explosion-implosion of selfhood that virtual reproduction has instigated. Intention matters and still affects social media representations of selfhood, but it seems that one pertinent consequence of social media's effects on identity is that it is distancing us from intentionality—we are, instead, becoming part of the machine of social media technology, and it works through us in a way that makes it just as much a user of us as we are of it. The speed at which we are able to construct our social media identities in fragments, with little thought or deliberation, is part of the slipping away of intentionality, but even more than this, the media itself gives us everything, and too much of everything, literally at our fingertips. Unlike a professional photographer, whose training and vocation promote caution, deliberateness, and intentionality, a person who takes a photo on a smartphone and posts it to social media *can* do so without caution, thought, or deliberation; this does not mean that he or she will do this, but it makes action without thought more accessible. On the surface, it seems there is a noble element in making the art of virtual identity construction available and accessible equally to everyone, but beneath the surface of this is corporate intentions and profits. The technology discourages thought and caution in those who are complacent, encouraging its users to acquiesce to user-friendliness and ease of access. However, we can combat the tendencies of complacency that it encourages by becoming more thoughtful and critical of our own behaviors.

The media is not simply part of the construction and representation of our individual identities; we are part of the media's construction and representation of its own identity—as the media is a product in a consumerist market. Social media companies want us to engage in the cloning of selfhood in order to create identification dependency in us. So now, where we might in the past have shared good news about an award or the birth of a child by word of mouth or an announcement in a monthly newsletter, we have the ability to share our personal news instantly and globally. The line between self and others is diminished, just as is the line between news and everyday life. Everything has become news, and as we are part of the mass reproduction of images of news, news is becoming a space for selfhood and personal identity assertion. Because of social media, what we eat for dinner and where we're going tomorrow is news—news that is not filtered and that pops up right alongside weather news from official sources; the trivialities of our personal lives constitute social media news so that we all feel a sense of the possibility of mattering, even though our popularity with the audience of our identities determines the reaction we receive in asserting our identity, which might either be nothing at all or something quite spectacular and absurd.

As 24/7 reporters on the scene of our selfhood, we are faced with both our agency and our confusion over how to direct or modify rapidly developing changes to our self-representations and self-concepts. Many individuals struggle with the effects of social media on their lives, particularly the damage it incurs on their sense of personhood and their ability to separate themselves from it. We eat, sleep, and breathe social media. Our phones are with many of us from the time we wake up until the time we fall asleep; sometimes they are on our bellies while we sleep. This, inevitably, is affecting the way we think—especially the way we think about ourselves because social media is all about "the self," constructing it and distributing it. Are we being cloned? Are we cloning our "selves"? Yes and no. According to Benjamin, "technical reproduction can put the copy of the original into situations which would be out of reach for the original itself,"[4] but when social media distributes a copy of an image of our authentic selfhood (our original self), it is not putting out an exact copy of it; it is only distributing an exact copy of a fragment of it. Social media images, such as those displayed on Facebook profiles and posts, are clones, and not always exact clones, of the particles of selfhood—not of selfhood itself. Identity can be constructed in words, behaviors, or in virtual technologies, but it is more complicated than that. We can only know identity in fragments, not in wholes. This is something we don't need social media to understand but about which we can remind ourselves in our engagements with social media technologies. Social media may clone images of us, but it will never clone *us*.

Facebook recently issued an announcement to its users that, due to a virus, information about some of its users had been leaked, the result of which was the cloning of accounts. Due to this leaking of information, user account information was copied, exactly, and reproduced for questionable purposes. Instead of one "John Smith from Nova Scotia," there might have been two—bearing the exact likeness in profile information, including photographic representation. The result could have been that friends of the original-virtual "Joe Schmoe from Nova Scotia" might receive friend-requests from the cloned (or fake) "Joe Schmoe from Nova Scotia." And "Joe Schmoe from Nova Scotia (the First)" might even receive a friend request from his clone, "Joe Schmoe from Nova Scotia (the Second)," the result of which might have been confusion, chaos, a bit of laughter, or, for gullible friends who clicked on a link offered by the clone of Joe Schmoe 1, the acquisition of a virus that would result in the cloning of their accounts and a replication of the process. One might argue, based on this Facebook cloning hoax phenomenon, that the cloning of selfhood is, indeed, happening before our eyes, but what's actually happening is the cloning of the image, not the self. And this distinction is a helpful reminder to us of the necessary separation that should be maintained between social media representation and personal identity, because without a sense of separation, we might deprive ourselves of critical inquiry into our identities. We must remind ourselves that we are more than our social media representations, that we are beings capable of introspection; but this becomes harder and harder to do, given our dependence on technology and how integrated our ideas of our selves have become with our virtual representations of our selves. If "Joe Schmoe (the First)" has a Twitter account or Snapchat account, in addition to his Facebook account, then he surely is engaging in the bifurcation of his virtual identity, which could have real repercussions on the way he sees himself and considers his identity. In some instances, if he is a critical thinker, it might expand and develop his idea of himself, but in others, it might lead him to see himself more as a fixed image or self than as a person capable of developing his ideas and identity at all times. There may be six virtual versions of one "Joe Schmoe from Nova Scotia (the First)" but there is only one individual behind those virtual representations. Just as there may be a thousand clones, in name only, of "Joe Schmoe," those clones affect our collective concept of what it means to be "Joe Schmoe"; but the cloning of the name—or the identity—alone does not equate with the cloning of the individual.

Establishing a sense of the separation between self and selfhood-representation is a compartmentalization that could be beneficial in establishing and maintaining a sense of identity away from social media. Social media users undoubtedly think of themselves differently because of their social media uses: their psychic monologue is affected by their virtual engagements and interactions just as much as their virtual engagements and interactions are affected by their psychic monologue. This reciprocity demonstrates the impact of social media on the self, as well as the slippery relationship between virtual and actual life. Many social media users would argue that virtual life is part of actual life, and it's hard to argue that it's not, given that the reality is that millions of people spend much of their time in front of computers and are active on social media technology.

From Liberating Second Lives to the Dead Ends of Catfishers, Trolls, and Twits

Many would also argue that spending one's life in a virtual reality is just as valid, if not more valid, than spending it in actual reality, that a virtual reality is an actual reality, and that the metaphysical connections made on social media are just as—if not more—fulfilling and substantial as those made in physical life. These are valid opinions with lived experience to back them up, but they are perspectives that should be explored further. No form of social media technology better exemplifies this outlook than the online virtual media application known as Second Life. The program, which dubs itself an "online virtual world," involves the construction of an identity and life that is virtual: it allows users to create identities, to establish connections (relationships and families), and to engage in any kind of life behavior in which they wish to engage—virtually. Users are limited to the regions of the virtual world to which they can travel, depending on how much they are willing to pay. They can pay to create a self that represents them according to their wishes; they can go to a virtual store that allows them to buy not only clothing but also skin. They can seek out virtual plastic surgery if they wish, but they must do so with real money. They can go to a certain virtual island and build a bungalow there, but they must pay real money to do so. And so, just as the virtual and actual worlds of the user collide in using the "virtual world," which its developers deny is a game, so too do the virtual and actual collide in the commoditizing of identity. A user of Second Life can be who he or she wants to be, but only virtually—and always for a price.

Questions of the ethics of virtual exploitation for profit need to be raised, but there are additional questions that must also be raised, especially regarding the impact that a virtual reality as elaborate as Second Life is having on actual people. Second Life allows users to chat in writing or vocally, while simulating graphic virtual acts. If two actual individuals, for instance, engage in virtual romantic or sexual acts, over a course of time, are the actual individuals invested or culpable or do the effects of these acts only have an impact in the virtual realm, not outside of it? It is obvious that engaging in a virtual sex act, like engaging in phone sex, has physical repercussions that extend beyond the virtual context, but, aside from physical manifestations of physical pleasure derived from visual and psychic stimulation, what else is happening? Second Life provides a prime example of the conflation of virtual and actual identity.

Avatars, as an extension of personhood, affect our minds. When we engage repeatedly in living a virtual "second life" as an avatar, we might lose our ability to draw the necessary line between reality and fantasy, if we are not careful, just as a public figure might be unable to draw the line between his or her public image and private life. Such engagements demand the suspension of disbelief. They also require that individuals are able to tell the difference between reality and fantasy, but social media technologies like Second Life are blurring that line for people who are susceptible, such as those who live isolated lives and those whose actual lives are not accurate representations of their interior selves. For a closeted lesbian in an unhappy marriage to a man, for instance, Second Life might provide some life-saving psychic relief, but that is precisely because of the bifurcation of her identity that hiding her desires (or "real self") causes. The relief of the ability to express real desires via the fantasy, partially lived out in the virtual world, is not liberation; it is an act of desperation, a survival mechanism, one that could save a life but not necessarily transform the life toward a state of greater authenticity. In some instances, a virtual lesbian relationship on Second Life might help the closeted lesbian to actualize her desires, establish her identity, and live a more authentic life (via a divorce from her husband in real life). On the other hand, if she is unable to manage living two lives, she might end up suffering mental or physical consequences that could be severe. For instance, if she tries to actualize a virtual relationship that she believes is significant in her life, she might end up in trouble—the individual on the other end of the virtual relationship may not be ready for that actualization, which could lead to legal or other consequences if the boundaries are not accepted. The answer is not to destroy or regulate virtual programs that sometimes play a role in disastrous situations; the answer is to self-regulate, to be critical and careful, and to understand both ourselves and the technologies we are using well enough to protect ourselves from harm.

The trouble with virtual technology is that in allowing us to construct our identities, it allows us to represent or misrepresent our "selves." Sometimes what appears to be misrepresentation (a girl using a selfie app that makes her look like a wolf) is actually representation (the girl is expressing her inner nature, which she sees as a pack animal). But sometimes what appears to be representation is misrepresentation, as in the case of an elderly man posing as a young man in order to trick a young girl into sending him nude photos of herself or agreeing to meet him in Central Park. Twitter, a virtual medium known for its succinct platform for communication, has become a virtual breeder of bot accounts and anonymous accounts. In addition to allowing for the creation of accounts without actual users attached to them, thousands of Twitter users choose to remain anonymous. Anonymity on Twitter happens for a variety of reasons, but sometimes it happens because people wish to communicate with or harass someone—or trick someone they know or do not know in real life into communicating with them. In other instances, users create accounts posing as someone they are not in order to attract attention or in order to manipulate another person into communicating with them.

Catfishing, a term used to describe the deceptive act of luring someone into communication or a relationship under the false pretense of a fake online persona, is becoming more and more popular, particularly on sites like Twitter that allow for and encourage anonymity. Despite the benefits of virtual anonymity, such as freedom of expression and the resistance against censorship and tyranny, the risks of virtual anonymity should be taken into consideration because the damage it potentially causes can be extreme. At the same time that anonymity suggests protection and preservation of the self against criticism or harm, it also allows for anonymous acts of harm to occur against vulnerable individuals. Social media users who expose information about their actual selves, especially on Twitter, need to be cautious about what anonymous others might be doing with that information. But anonymous accounts are not the only threat to safe virtual identity-making practices: highly constructed identities representing actual people can be just as dangerous. Consider the example of the use of social media by persons in power, particularly the presidential use of Tweets by Donald Trump, who frequently uses the medium to throw tantrums and express himself, often demonstrating very little insight in his Twitter outbursts. Twitter and other sites allow for ranting, raving, and raging, much of which can be healthy and critical, but they also allow for the construction of identities that are solely based on these one-dimensional sound bites of selfhood, and this can be to the detriment of critical discourse, not to mention international dialogue and diplomacy.

Virtual identity making is personal and political, and the way we represent ourselves affects the way we see ourselves and the way that others see us. The effect of social media on identity is different for each individual, and the benefits and risks depend on the individual, but we should all be asking questions about representation, as it is undeniable that our lives and our identities are becoming enmeshed with the technologies with which we engage. Our self-concepts and our minds are being affected by our virtual navigation of the self. While our individual intentions in using social media technology may be good, we cannot simply trust the technology to be good to us, or for us, in return.

Authentic selfhood and virtual selfhood do more than coexist; they become integrated, mostly via the integration of virtual selfhood into the self-concept of the living being. When people take selfies, they see themselves. They have the opportunity to influence the reproduced images of their authentic presence in time and space through the photo, and they also have the opportunity to manipulate and distort these images. The construction of virtual identity is having an impact on our material identities and real lives—for instance, the vortex of time we enter into when we "browse" through and become psychically inundated with images of art, religion, film, food, and other commodities serves as a consumerist gray space: we are partial-consumers, consuming images of material goods mentally but not physically. We assume that we are engaging with ideas and storing them up while not also realizing that we are engaging with virtual consumerism. But what's at stake in terms of cultural capital? The commodification of our identities and our consciousnesses is at stake. This is not a revelation, but we have not yet adequately navigated and philosophized the potency and ramifications attached to social media's commodification of identity. The virtual element exacerbates, distorts, and renders unclear the nature and effects of this commodification.

What we share on social media platforms simultaneously shapes and reflects how we identify holistically, and we become psychically consumed with the act of identifying with consumerist images that are marketed as tools for the expression of personal interests and preferences. If we compartmentalize in relating to social media sites, we are not necessarily better off than if we go with the flow between virtual and physical reality, but either way, and whether we take this to be of positive or negative consequence, the way we think is undeniably affected. By categorizing consumerist images that represent our "selves" on social media sites, we are also rearranging the internal categories we hold about what we like, what we do, and who we are.

Mirroring the loss of origin on Pinterest, Facebook, Twitter, and other sites on which material is shared, often with no reference point; our preferences and the identifications of others meld with our own in such a way that, without critical thought, it is possible for us to lose a sense of where they came from or how they formed. To try to trace an image on Pinterest, for example, to the original board on which it was pinned is not impossible, but Pinterest does not make it easy. In much the same way, social media technology does not make it easy for us to be introspective about our use of it or to trace back the formation of our identities within it. The images, like fragments from a lost history, usurp or mask the context in which the images arise—and our identities, formed by them, are difficult to identify and describe because they have developed so rapidly and completely, enshrouding us in representations without a sense of origin for, or attachments to, those representations. Our identities are being consumed by virtual consumerism; consumerism is becoming internalized in us in new ways—ways that may make us more or less materially entrenched in it and culpable for its effects within and around us. What is unique about this is that we recognize in bits and pieces what is happening to us, collectively, but we remain helpless. Despite our awareness of the uselessness of applying an old logic to a situation to which it cannot and never will apply, we have trouble developing a new logic and applying it.

There are significant trade-offs to the alternate consciousness options that 21st-century social media provide. With the rise of social media and the birth of new psychical realities, we are seeing the decline of physical activity and relating. Social media has created a converse relationship between physicality and psychicality. Although the mind and body should not be considered separate entities, social media technology is, indeed, affecting the way we experience them: "mind-body" is becoming more and more disconnected in the same way that our growing global connections online are increasingly accompanied by declining intimacy and physical connection between ourselves and those in closest proximity to us.

Psychicality is virtually replacing physicality when it comes to identity, representation, and relation in certain parts of our lives, and there are consequences to this of which we are only remotely aware. Invested fully in our alternate realities, we have become divested of our former senses of reality, but how deep into this rabbit hole can we go before we begin to recognize our new selves and understand them in relation to our old selves? Social media technology has launched us into a new consciousness and new sense-making, for better or worse, and it is imperative that we begin to engage in studies of our technoselves in order to try to articulate this metaphorically death-and-life situation as it unfolds within and around us, despite how confusing it is and how little of it we are equipped to comprehend.

We are, like Alice, on an adventure in the identity wonderland of social media, experiencing our identities differently according to individual virtual situations, but hopefully with a sense of curiosity and a determination to make sense, even if we must understand sense in new ways in order to do it. Every person who engages with social media technology is experiencing a second set of circumstances through which to experience life and identity, but there is only one life that we live, virtually or physically. There may be a virtual game called Second Life, but there is no second life. Will we, like Alice at the end of her dream, wake up from virtual reality to reality, or has our sense of reality been permanently altered by the ways social media technologies have expanded our consciousness? If we are critical thinkers—as critical as we are curious and full of wonder—we will have the opportunity to wake up, not from a virtual reality, but to a reality of identity that is both virtual and physical.

Notes

1. Paul Valery, "The Conquest of Ubiquity," in David Thorburn, Henry Jenkins, and Edward Barrett, eds., *Rethinking Media Change: The Aesthetics of Transition* (Cambridge, MA: The MIT Press, 2004).

2. Walter Benjamin, "The Work of Art in the Age of Its Technological Reproducibility," in Michael W. Jennings, Brigid Doherty, and Thomas Y. Levin, eds., *The Work of Art in the Age of Its Technological Reproducibility, and Other Writings on Media 2008* (Cambridge, MA: Belknap Press, 2008).

3. Ibid.

4. Ibid.

CHAPTER TEN

Deep Fakes and Computer Vision: The Paradox of New Images

Lisa Portmess

We believe that Google should not be in the business of war.
—Letter by more than 4,000 employees
protesting Project Maven, 2018

Image files therefore leave no trail, and it is often impossible to establish with certainty the provenance of a digital image.
—William Mitchell, *The Reconfigured Eye:*
Visual Truth in the Post-Photographic Era, 1992

So that often, in order to be more perfect as images and to represent an object better, they must not resemble it.
—René Descartes, *Optics*, 1637

In April 2017, the U.S. Department of Defense established Project Maven to draw on advanced AI technology created in the private sector to interpret high-resolution aerial images gathered from drone surveillance. Known as the Algorithmic Warfare Cross-Functional Team, Project Maven employs computer vision techniques for object recognition and classification derived from the full motion visual data gathered from drone footage. Technology developed for Project Maven has been deployed by the U.S. military's Middle East and Africa commands and is now being developed for use in high-altitude surveillance aircraft, enemy target assessment, and analysis of captured material.[1] Project Maven is the first known application of sophisticated AI in combat zones, giving rise to intense ethical debates about the development and use of machine learning in war with its biologically inspired neural networks adapted for military use. As a result of protests against Project Maven by more than 4,000 employees in April 2018, Google agreed not to renew its contract with the Pentagon that is up for renewal in 2019. Critics contend that the weaponization of AI signals movement toward lethally autonomous machines and "killer robots" and risks a global arms race. Its defenders emphasize its utility in providing comprehensive image processing from aerial surveillance, which will help to reduce civilian and military casualties through greater precision in targeting in war-fighting environments. Algorithmic warfare has intensified international debate over whether such fully autonomous weapons systems can comply with international humanitarian law and human rights law.[2] Key to such compliance is the capacity to discern morally significant differences in identified objects of military interest such as the distinction between combatants and noncombatants.

Project Maven is not the only such AI program directed at enhancing military surveillance and target recognition. JEDI, a Joint Enterprise Defense Initiative, is a $10 billion cloud acquisition project projected to consolidate infrastructure and enhance war-fighting capacity through more efficient exploitation of information.[3] Tech companies such as Amazon Web Services, Oracle, and IBM are expected to bid, with the winner announced in spring 2019. Facing internal revolt from its employees, Google announced just before the bidding process ended in October 2018 that it had withdrawn its bid for the contract. The ethical debate over Project Maven has proved complex. Google officials at first claimed that Project Maven was not "offensive" in nature. With deep unease over drone counterinsurgency warfare and the high rate of civilian casualties, ethical concern over Project Maven has intensified over its potential for sophisticated targeting capacity of human subjects. With the Pentagon making artificial intelligence a central feature of its weapons strategy for the future, algorithmic warfare is now at the center of debates over autonomous weapons systems and their relationship to human decision making.

This chapter explores the relationship of artificial intelligence with counterinsurgency and counterterrorism efforts and examines philosophical analysis of digital image processing and its relevance to digital maps that annotate objects of military interest and improve recognition and tracking. Paradoxically, such images generated by machine-learning algorithms, which are meant to enhance image understanding and enhance our grasp of reality, share the same uncertain ontology with computer-generated digital impersonation and deep fakes used in malicious hoaxes and fake news. This paper examines this parallel and argues that *new images* and their enabling technologies require rethinking the nature of digital image processing in high-stakes war-fighting contexts in which authentication is rarely possible and ethical issues remain intractable.

Algorithmic Warfare and Lethality: Ethical Arguments

Amid intense debate over the role of AI and machine learning in modern warfare among policy makers, ethicists, scientists and military planners, the ethical arguments expressed by Google employees against Project Maven are focused on the lethality of fully autonomous weapons with the power to target and deploy without human control. Such arguments are intensified by a more general concern over the relationship of tech companies to the U.S. military in the transfer of war-fighting technologies. Protesters emphasize Google's responsibility to abide by its core values and its motto, Don't Be Evil. "We believe that Google should not be in the business of war."[4] Neither, protesters argue, should Google, with its worldwide mission, affiliate with any one nation's military, contribute to the possible acceleration of algorithmic warfare, or outsource the moral responsibility of our technologies to third parties. Humans, not algorithms, should be responsible for the potentially lethal work of identifying enemy targets and should refuse to assist the U.S. government in military surveillance with potentially lethal outcomes.[5] The letter concludes by demanding the company "draft, publicize, and enforce a clear policy stating that neither Google nor its contractors will ever build warfare technology." In an open letter of support for Google employees and tech workers, the International Committee For Robot Arms Control (ICRAC) issued a letter of solidarity from scholars, academics, and researchers urging Google to support efforts to ban autonomous weapons and commit to not developing military technologies.[6] ICRAC urged that Google pledge neither to participate nor support the development, manufacture, trade, or use of autonomous weapons.

Ethical concern has also been voiced about risks that AI will contribute to perpetual war by giving some of the most powerful tech companies a stake in perpetuating such wars and bringing big tech companies more deeply into the military-industrial complex.[7] The Pentagon's AI projects have dramatically increased with the establishment of the Joint Artificial Intelligence Center (JAIC), which will oversee approximately 600 AI projects at easily $1.7 billion. In September 2018 the Defense Advanced Research Projects Agency (DARPA) announced its plan to invest up to $2 billion in AI weapons research:

> The problem isn't the quality of the tools, in other words, but the institution wielding them. And AI will only make that institution more brutal. The forever war demands that the US sees enemies everywhere. AI promises to find those enemies faster—even if all it takes to be considered an enemy is exhibiting a pattern of behavior that a (classified) machine-learning model associates with hostile activity.[8]

Still another concern is expressed by Miles Brundage of the Future of Humanity Institute in his report, "The Malicious Use of Artificial Intelligence: Forecasting, Prevention and Mitigation." The report examines potential security threats from malicious uses of AI technologies, and recommends ways to forecast, prevent and mitigate such threats.

> We expect novel attacks that subvert cyberphysical systems (e.g. causing autonomous vehicles to crash) or involve physical systems that it would be infeasible to direct remotely (e.g. a swarm of thousands of micro-drones). The use of AI to automate tasks involved in surveillance (e.g. analyzing mass-collected data), persuasion (e.g. creating targeted propaganda), and deception (e.g. manipulating videos) may expand threats associated with privacy invasion and social manipulation.[9]

Because AI systems suffer from unresolved vulnerabilities, no system can be fully protected from malicious use. These include such harms as "data poisoning attacks (introducing training data that causes a learning system to make mistakes), adversarial examples (designed to be misclassified by machine learning systems), and the exploitation of flaws in the design of autonomous systems' goals."[10] In addition, the possession of unresolved vulnerabilities increases the possibility of attacks that specifically exploit these vulnerabilities:

> If multiple robots are controlled by a single AI system run on a centralized server, or if multiple robots are controlled by identical AI systems and presented with the same stimuli, then a single attack could also produce simultaneous failures on an otherwise implausible scale. A worst-case scenario in this category might be an attack on a server used to direct

autonomous weapon systems, which could lead to large-scale friendly fire or civilian targeting.[11]

As these arguments indicate, algorithmic warfare reveals the disruptive power of new technologies, where long experience has yet to be brought to bear in meaningful attempts to mitigate risks. These risks involve not only the subversion of servers and the hacking of data but also risks that arise from a more fundamental vulnerability of image-processing algorithms to unpredictability and inexplicable decision making. Most urgent are the ethical concerns that focus on whether lethal autonomous warfare can meet ethical standards and conform to the laws of war and whether they can be given failsafe controls to assure protection from cyberattacks.

Peter W. Singer, strategist and fellow at New American and author of *Wired for War: The Robotics Revolution and Conflict in the 21st Century* and *Like War: The Mechanization of Social Media*, views the mechanization of warfare as a long, steady trajectory with increasingly greater autonomy embedded in war-fighting technologies, even in wars with their ancillary social media battlefields driven by Twitter bots.[12] He notes:

> Humans started moving out of "the loop" of war long before robots made their way onto battlefields. As far back as World War II, the Norden bombsight made calculations of height, speed, and trajectory too complex for a human to automatically decide when to drop a bomb on a B-17 and antipersonnel landmines once planted exploded autonomously and indiscriminately.[13]

At sea the Aegis computer system was developed in the 1980s, operating in four systems of increasing autonomy to defend U.S. Navy ships from aerial attack. Singer observes that "it is not that the Matrix or Cylons are taking over, but rather that a redefinition of what it means to have humans 'in the loop' of decision making has long been under way, with the authority and autonomy of machines ever expanding."[14]

In a *New York Times* interview, Singer notes that "many of the tools that the Pentagon was seeking were neither strictly military nor strictly civilian."[15] Software that can be used for military purposes can also be used to track movement at factory distribution centers, suggesting that the boundary between technologies of civilian and military use are too porous for clear distinction. Singer also notes that Google's search engine and the video platform of its YouTube division have been used by warriors of many countries as well as by Islamic warfighters and Al Qaeda. Google employees may want to act like they're not in the business of war, he remarks, but the war long ago came to them. For Singer, this realism is not to undermine the need for political, ethical, legal, and economic discussion over how wars are fought and who fights them but rather to highlight the complexity and long trajectory of automated war-fighting technologies and the military-civilian cooperation that has produced them. Algorithms are likely to become the conceptual and technological foundation for future war-fighting, and "advice provided by algorithms" and the advice is likely to become a significant determinant of future military judgments.[16] Like all systems in dynamic environments, there is reason for caution in how such advice should be taken, emerging as it does from machine learning with unpredictable forms of rationality not our own and from susceptibilities to cyberattacks and other hostile interference by adversaries.

Digital Images, Algorithmic Uncertainties

The ontology of photographs has long preoccupied philosophers interested in the nature of the photograph and what was widely believed to be its superiority of object representation. The photograph was understood to be an image chemically and optically brought into being by the objects in the world it captures. The photograph was thought to carry the imprint of the real even when the possibility of photographic manipulation was understood. New images, digitally produced, had not yet arisen when many of the seminal texts in photography were written. Yet the concern for the ontology of the photograph has persisted even with the rise of digitally produced images and their fluid, less certain relationship to what they represent. Versions of these philosophical and aesthetic questions have found their way into discussions of digital image processing and algorithmic warfare, where concerns about cybersecurity and the protection of data is of highest concern. A brief exploration of the debate over the ontology of the photograph clarifies the reasons for concern over the nature of *new images* that are digitally produced.

In his article "The Ontology of Digital Photographs and Images," Koray Degirmenci observes that photography involves a complex relationship between an image and its referent in that the object being photographed is effectively etched on the photographic surface, a property of photographs he terms "indexicality," where the photographic surface is an index of the actual object being photographed.[17] Reflecting on the "ineradicable fragility of our ontological distinctions between the imaginary and the real," Degirmenci examines how computer-manipulated imagery appears to threaten the truth value of photography even after decades of semiotic analysis emphasize the "image-idea." Yet it is not the uncertainty of any single digital photograph only that is unsettling, he argues, but rather the prospect that any photograph might be digitally altered. Digital alteration undermines faith in the transparency of the photograph and threatens the subject's position in the act of perception, raising concerns about the automation of vision in digital image processing and machine learning.

Even before the emergence of digital photography, critical attention was given to the role of photography as one of mediation rather than reflection of the real. Philosophers of technology and critical theorists emphasized the active role of the technological artifact of the camera in shaping perception. With its framing limitations and its temporal finitude, the camera determines the photograph as much as the object photographed. The eye of the photographer was understood as bringing into being an image of the world as perceived rather than replicating the real. Still, the belief that the photograph carried the trace of the real kept its hold and set the standard for the documentary impact that attaches still to the photographic image and certifies presence at a certain place and time. This confidence in photographic verification has brought surveillance cameras and police cams to public spaces and created a continuous flow of surveillance data intended to capture real events in time. Even with evidence of the ambiguity of surveillance images and the tendency of interpreters to perceive ambiguous stimuli in ways that reflect prior beliefs, confidence remains strong in photographic verification and the idea of a neutral image.

Image-processing AI with machine learning is developing in this context of high confidence in photographic verification, appealing not only to commercial uses such as self-driving cars but to the need in war-fighting environments to process high volumes of surveillance data at tremendous velocity with comprehensive attention to detail. Yet amid this confidence is a growing realization of the contradictory mix of properties of digital images that are "simultaneously powerful and brittle, brilliant and childlike, dazzling and incomprehensible."[18] Their properties are not the properties of past programmable machines. It is not fully understood what AI machine-learning processes have learned or how they categorize data. This uncertainty is heightened in neural network machines that evolve in real time. Such emergent behavior renders digital processing and its rationality fundamentally unknowable.

Digital image processing depends on the instructions and rules that algorithms use to interpret data, yet the algorithmic conversion of such data to usable outputs is affected by feedback loops or recursion, in which data collected for algorithm training has real-world responses fed back to the algorithm. Feedback loops are implicated in algorithmic bias and compound the bias that can arise from underlying social and institutional ideologies that affect the design of software and the input of training data. Algorithms used in digital image processing are poised to play a critical role in the conceptual analysis of surveillance data, in which object recognition and classification are dependent not on neutral image processing but on algorithms, themselves human artifacts that reflect their fallible human creators.

With the advent of digital imaging techniques in the early 1990s, philosophical attention grappled with the revolution in the production of the photographic image. The more fluid relationship of the digital image to the real thing imaged challenged notions of the photograph as an indexical sign and raised questions about whether a digital image could be said to be an image in the traditional sense. A digital photo is created by cameras that contain electronic photodetectors that capture images focused by a lens, as opposed to an exposure on photographic film. Unlike analog photographs, created by physical signs and marks on particular surfaces, the digital medium does not relay physical properties. Instead it transforms information, symbolizing physical properties mathematically by arbitrary numerical codes, with "reversible and convertible characteristics" and no "certificate of evidence (and presence)" as analog photographs are believed to have.[19] Yet the paradox of digital photography, according to Lev Manovich, is in the way it imitates the cultural and aesthetic codes of analog photography. He argues provocatively that digital imagery "annihilates photography while solidifying, glorifying and immortalizing the photographic." The photograph is a certificate of presence of a thing and carries traces of it where the trace of the digital image is "lost after the very brief moment of the actual photographic act."[20] He states:

> Most of the historically important functions of the human eye are being supplanted by practices in which visual images no longer have any reference to the position of an observer in a "real," optically perceived world. If these images can be said to refer to anything, it is to millions of bits of electronic mathematical data. Increasingly visuality will be situated on a cybernetic and electromagnetic terrain where abstract visual and linguistic elements coincide and are consumed, circulated, and exchanged globally.[21]

Coming to terms with digital images requires recognizing the disruptive impact of digital images and the fluid, undefined relationship these images have to their referents. In *The Reconfigured Eye*, William J. Mitchell writes:

> There is simply no equivalent of the permanently archived, physically unique photographic negative. Image files are ephemeral, can be copied and transmitted virtually instantly and cannot be examined (as photographic negative can) for physical evidence of tampering. The only difference between an original file and a copy is the tag recording time and date of creation, and that can easily be changed. Image files therefore leave no trail, and it is often impossible to establish with certainty the provenance of a digital image.[22]

Mitchell's observation has proven astute with the increasing presence online of deep fakes and other forms of digital impersonation that threaten democratic governments by destabilizing elections and information environments with sophisticated AI-engendered fake news.

Skepticism about the ontology of the digital image is expressed well by Peter Benson in "The Ontology of Photography: From Analogue to Digital," subtitled "On Why Digital Photos Aren't Reliable Records of Anything." To see something as a digital image, he argues, is to place it within the category of simulacra, a distinctive category of objects. The proliferation of digital images blurs the distinction between the domain of the photograph and its relation to the real with the domain of the digital images. "We are never quite sure what kind of image we are seeing. And it is in this sense that digital photography contributes to our ontological uncertainty."[23] Benson cites Barthes, who believes the essence of perceiving something as a photograph can be summed up in the phrase "that has been": "In photography," Barthes writes, "I can never deny that the thing has been there."[24] We should be concerned, Benson argues, about the replacement of traditional photography by digital images "before the final vestiges of reality vanish."[25] The phenomenon of deep fakes, an AI-based human image synthesis technique, is one such pressing concern over lost vestiges of reality that bear, unexpectedly, on national security and, more deeply, on how we perceive the world.

Fake videos and digital impersonation have become commonplace on the Internet and are a source of urgent concern for scholars, information analysts, military experts, and governments. Deep fakes, used to create fake news and malicious hoaxes, are made possible by advances in deep-learning algorithms that synthesize audio and video content that is highly realistic, depicting real people speaking and acting in ways that they have never spoken or acted.[26] Some concerns are as follows:

As this technology spreads, the ability to produce bogus yet credible video and audio content will come within the reach of an ever-larger array of governments, nonstate actors, and individuals. As a result, the ability to advance lies using hyperrealistic, fake evidence is poised for a great leap forward. A well-timed and thoughtfully scripted deep fake or series of deep fakes could tip an election, spark violence in a city primed for civil unrest, bolster insurgent narratives about an enemy's supposed atrocities, or exacerbate political divisions in a society. The opportunities for the sabotage of rivals are legion—for example, sinking a trade deal by slipping to a foreign leader a deep fake purporting to reveal the insulting true beliefs or intentions of U.S. officials.[27]

Such manipulation is a matter of global as well as national security attention by those tracking the malicious uses of artificial intelligence and the risks to emerging AI projects such as Project Maven.[28] The U.S. Defense Department is consulting with outside experts on detection and prevention of fake videos, concerned with the national security implications of the spread of misinformation through manipulated audio and video. Deep fake technology contributes to an already sophisticated array of disinformation that interacts with a vulnerable information environment, a "seeing is believing" trust in the authenticity of the image, and biases that diminish skepticism.

The risks of deep fake technologies are not particular to Project Maven. As algorithmic warfare moves beyond defensive systems such as cyber and antimissile defense, its conceptual and technical power, its rapid decision making, and its alternative rationality are likely to have a profound effect on war-fighting, intensifying ethical concerns. Such ethical concern, already acute over algorithmic bias in image recognition technologies, focuses on the technical limitations in design as well as the explicit or implicit biases in the systemic coding, collecting, and selection of data used to train algorithms. Image-recognition technologies with machine learning play an increasingly sophisticated role in knowledge acquisition and shape not only what we see but also how it appears to us. Because of the intertwined relationship of technology with knowledge acquisition, image-recognition technologies inevitably disrupt and create new forms of mediated perception that will require a wide array of authentication and interpretive responses, as well as efforts at technological solutions, effective criminal penalties, regulatory action, and law and public policy responses.[29] It is vital that the digital image be seen as a site of contested meaning.

Conclusion

New images and their enabling technologies require rethinking the nature of digital image processing in high-risk contexts of algorithmic warfare, where authentication is rarely possible and ethical issues are intractable. Images are neither transparent nor legible without interpretation, and the risks of indiscriminate killings, inherent in banned weapons such as landmines, cluster bombs, and chemical weapons, are heightened in algorithmic warfare by the uncertain state of truth in the digital image and its fluid and precarious relationship to the real.

Notes

1. Cheryl Pellerin, "Project Maven to Deploy Computer Algorithms to War Zone by Year's End," *U.S. Department of Defense*, July 21, 2017, https://dod .defense.gov/News/Article/Article/1254719/project-maven-to-deploy-computer -algorithms-to-war-zone-by-years-end/.

2. Ted Piccone, "How Can International Law Regulate Autonomous Weapons?" *Brookings Institute*, April 10, 2018, https://www.brookings.edu/blog/order-from -chaos/2018/04/10/how-can-international-law-regulate-autonomous-weapons/.

3. Lisa Ferdinando, "Officials Highlight Role of Cloud Infrastructure in Supporting Warfighters," *U.S. Department of Defense*, March 14, 2018, https://dod .defense.gov/News/Article/Article/1466699/dod-officials-highlight-role-of-cloud -infrastructure-in-supporting-warfighters/.

4. Letter to Google CEO Sundar Pichai, April 2018.

5. Kate Conger, "Google Employees Resign in Protest against Google Contract," *Gizmodo*, May 4, 2016.

6. "Open Letter in Support of Google Employees and Tech Workers," *International Committee for Robot Arms Control*, June 25, 2018, https://www.icrac.net /open-letter-in-support-of-google-employees-and-tech-workers/.

7. Ben Tarnoff, "Weaponized AI Is Coming. Are Algorithmic Forever Wars Our Future?" *Guardian*, October 11, 2018, https://www.theguardian.com /commentisfree/2018/oct/11/war-jedi-algorithmic-warfare-us-military.

8. Ibid.

9. Miles Brundage, Shahar Avin, Jack Clark, Helen Toner, Peter Eckersley, Ben Garfinkel, Allan Dafoe, Paul Scharre, Thomas Zeitzoff, Bobby Filar, Hyrum Anderson, Heather Roff, Gregory C. Allen, Jacob Steinhardt, Carrick Flynn, Seán Ó hÉigeartaigh, Simon Beard, Haydn Belfield, Sebastian Farquhar, Clare Lyle, Rebecca Crootof, Owain Evans, Michael Page, Joanna Bryson, Roman Yampolskiy, and Dario Amodei, "The Malicious Use of Artificial Intelligence: Forecasting, Prevention and Mitigation," *Future of Humanity Institute* (Oxford, United Kingdom), February 2017, https://arxiv.org/ftp/arxiv/papers/1802/1802.07228.pdf.

10. Ibid.

11. Ibid.

12. Peter W. Singer and Emerson T. Brooking, *Like War: The Mechanization of Social Media* (Boston, MA: Eamon Dolan/Houghton Mifflin Harcourt, 2018).

13. Peter W. Singer, "In the Loop: Armed Robots and the Future of War," *Brookings Institution*, January 28, 2009, https://www.brookings.edu/articles /in-the-loop-armed-robots-and-the-future-of-war/.

14. Ibid.

15. Daisuke Wakabayashi and Scott Shane, "Google Will Not Renew Pentagon Contract That Upset Employees," *New York Times*, June 1, 2018.

16. Peter Layton, *Algorithmic Warfare: Applying Artificial Intelligence to Warfighting* (Canberra, BC: Air Power Development Centre, Department of Defence, 2018), http://airpower.airforce.gov.au/APDC/media/PDF-Files/Contemporary%20 AirPower/AP33-Algorithmic-Warfare-Applying-Artificial-Intelligence-to-Warf ighting.pdf.

17. Koray Degirmenci, "The Ontology of Digital Photographs and Images," *Art-Sanat*, no. 8 (2017): 554.

18. Peter Layton, iii.

19. Lev Manovich, "The Paradoxes of Digital Photography," in Liz Wells, ed., *Photography: A Critical Introduction* (London: Routledge, 2006), 311–44.

20. Ibid., 568.

21. Ibid., 558.

22. William J. Mitchell, *The Reconfigured Eye: Visual Truth in the Post-Photographic Era* (Cambridge, MA: MIT Press, 1992), 51.

23. Peter Benson, "The Ontology of Photography: From Analogue to Digital," *Philosophy Now* no. 95 (2013), pp. 18–21. https://philosophynow.org/issues/95 /The_Ontology_of_Photography_From_Analogue_To_Digital.

24. Ibid.

25. Ibid.

26. Robert Chesney and Danielle Citron, "Disinformation on Steroids: The Threat of Deep Fakes." *Council on Foreign Relations*, October 16, 2018, https:// www.cfr.org/report/deep-fake-disinformation-steroids.

27. Ibid.

28. Will Knight, "The State Department Has Produced the First Tools for Catching Deep Fakes," *MIT Technology Review*, August 7, 2018, https://www .technologyreview.com/s/611726/the-defense-department-has-produced -the-first-tools-for-catching-deepfakes/.

29. Robert Chesney and Danielle Keats Citron, "Deep Fakes: A Looming Challenge for Privacy, Democracy, and National Security," *107 California Law Review* (posted online July 14, 2018, forthcoming in *California Law Review* in 2019); University of Texas Law, Public Law Research Paper No. 692; University of Maryland Legal Studies Research Paper No. 2018-21, https://ssrn.com/abstract =3213954 or http://dx.doi.org/10.2139/ssrn.3213954.

About the Editor and Contributors

Editor

C. G. Prado, PhD, is professor emeritus in philosophy at Queen's University, Kingston, Ontario. He is a fellow of the Royal Society and has published 20 books and anthologies, including *America's Post-Truth Phenomenon: When Feelings and Opinions Trump Facts and Evidence*, editor (Praeger, 2018); *Social Media and Your Brain: Web-Based Communication Is Changing How We Think and Express Ourselves*, editor (Praeger, 2016); *Coping with Choices to Die* (2011); *Starting with Descartes* (2009); *Foucault's Legacy*, editor (2009); *Choosing to Die: Elective Death and Multiculturalism* (2008); and *Searle and Foucault on Truth* (2006). He has also contributed 12 chapters to anthologies and published 30 journal articles.

Contributors

Babette Babich, PhD, is professor of philosophy at Fordham University in New York City. Author of over 250 journal articles and book chapters, she has edited 14 collective volumes, including *Of David Hume's Of the Standard of Taste* (forthcoming) and *Hermeneutic Philosophies of Social Science* (2017), and has been executive editor of the journal *New Nietzsche Studies* since 1996. Her recent monographs include *The Hallelujah Effect: Music, Performance Practice and Technology* (2016) and *Un Politique Brisé. Le Souci d'Autrui, l'Humanisme, et les Juifs Chez Heidegger* (2016).

Chris Beeman, PhD, is associate professor in education at Brandon University, Manitoba. He teaches in the area of indigenous epistemologies and ontologies, specializing in understanding the philosophical underpinnings of learning through indigenous perspectives. Beeman's research entails connecting with wilder places and interpreting an autochthonous way of being. This may occur in travels through relatively wilder places or in long-term interactions with the world. Recent publications may be found in *Encounters in the Theory and History of Education, The Journal of Experiential Education*, and *Trumpter*. Earlier work includes the documentary film *Ancient Futures*.

Jason Hannan, PhD, is associate professor in the Department of Rhetoric and Communications at the University of Winnipeg. He is the editor of *Truth in the Public Sphere* (2016) and *Philosophical Profiles in the Theory of Communication* (2014). He has authored articles in the *European Journal of Communication, Communication Theory, Contemporary Pragmatism, Empedocles: European Journal for the Philosophy of Communication, Review of Communication*, and *Intellectual History Review*. Hannan's research interests include media and communication theory, rhetorical theory and criticism, posthumanism and critical animal studies, and bioethics and medical humanities. He is currently completing a book titled *Rational Agonism: Alasdair MacIntyre's Philosophy of Communication*.

Jessica Lowell Mason is a PhD student in global gender and sexuality studies at the New York State University at Buffalo. She has taught composition at Spoon River College, Carl Sandburg College, and Western Illinois University. Mason has worked for Shakespeare in Delaware Park, Ujima Theatre Co., Just Buffalo Literary Center, the Jewish Repertory Theatre, and Prometheus Books. In 2014, she was awarded the Gloria Anzaldúa Rhetorician Award by the Conference on College Composition and Communication. Her works have appeared in a number of journals, including *The Comstock Review, Lambda Literary, Gender Focus, Sinister Wisdom, Lavender Review, IthacaLit*, and *The Feminist Wire*. Mason is cofounder of the feminist mental health literacy organization Madwomen in the Attic.

Lawrie McFarlane, PhD, is a retired deputy minister who ran health, education, and treasury board departments in British Columbia and Saskatchewan. He represented Saskatchewan at the Uruguay round of GATT negotiations in Geneva. He and C. G. Prado coauthored a book on health policy, *The Best-Laid Plans: Health Care's Problems and Prospects* (2002). McFarlane has also contributed editorials to the *Journal of the Canadian Medical Association*: "Is a Perfect Storm Brewing on the Health Care Front?" (2004) and "Supreme Court Slaps For-Sale Sign on Medicare" (2005). He is currently a columnist and editorial writer with the *Victoria Times Colonist* and has been published in most of Canada's leading newspapers.

Lisa Menard has worked for the Queen's University Office of Advancement for over a dozen years and specializes in planning customized contributor relations with the university's top donors. Prior to her work at Queen's University, Menard's career was focused on work in the nonprofit sector in Ottawa, Ontario. Among her volunteer activities, she is a community outreach coordinator and manages multiple outreach programs each year to help families in need in Kingston, Ontario.

Jennifer Parks, PhD, is professor of philosophy and director of the undergraduate bioethics minor program at Loyola University. Her areas of specialization include health care ethics, feminist theory, and social philosophy. Parks authored *No Place Like Home? Feminist Ethics and Home Health Care* and coauthored *The Complete Idiot's Guide to Understanding Ethics* and *Ethics, Aging, and Society: The Critical Turn*. She also coedited *Bioethics in a Changing World*. She has published articles in *The Hastings Center Report, Bioethics, The Journal of Medical Ethics, Hypatia: A Journal of Feminist Philosophy*, and *The International Journal of Feminist Approach to Bioethics*. Parks has also contributed to several collections on assisted reproduction and aging and long-term care.

Rossana Pasquino, PhD, is currently associate professor at the Dipartimento di Ingegneria Chimica, dei Materiali e della Produzione Industriale, Università degli Studi di Napoli Federico II in Napoli, Italy. She teaches rheology and transport phenomena to students of chemical and biomedical engineering. Pasquino is recognized for her work in the rheology of complex fluids, especially in the use of rheology as a tool to detect morphology and microscopic properties. In her work around the world—in Belgium, Greece, Switzerland, and Canada—she has been involved in various aspects of the soft-matter world, with particular attention on the rheological properties of viscoelastic solutions, colloids, and polymers. Pasquino is also an accomplished wheelchair fencer and competes for Italy in the National Paralympic team, both with épée and sabre. She will soon start her quest for Olympic qualification for the Tokyo 2020 Games.

Lisa Portmess, PhD, is Bittinger chair of philosophy at Gettysburg College. She has published in *Ethics, Information Technology, Theoria, Peace and Justice Studies, The Canadian Journal of Learning and Technology, The Public Affairs Quarterly*, and *St. Andrew Studies in Philosophy and Public Affairs*. Her recent work on philosophy and technology has examined big data and its linguistic representation, UN peacekeeping ethics and technology, cyberwar and its moral ambiguity, and MOOCs and postcolonial knowledge. Portmess has served as a professor at the American University of Beirut and as an American Philosophical Association Congressional fellow. She has also been a resident fellow at the Centre for Philosophy and Public Affairs at St. Andrews University and a Fulbright scholar at the American University of Cairo.

Index